ALCOHOL AND REPRODUCTION

ALCOHOL AND REPRODUCTION
A BIBLIOGRAPHY

Compiled by Ernest L. Abel

GREENWOOD PRESS

WESTPORT, CONNECTICUT • LONDON, ENGLAND

Library of Congress Cataloging in Publication Data

Abel, Ernest L., 1943–
    Alcohol and reproduction.

    Includes index.
        1. Fetal alcohol syndrome—Bibliography.   2. Alcohol—
Physiological effect—Bibliography.   3. Generative
organs—Effect of drugs on—Bibliography.   I. Title.
[DNLM: 1.   Alcohol, Ethyl—Adverse effects—Bibliography.
2. Fetal alcohol syndrome—Bibliography.   3. Reproduc-
tion—Drug effects—Bibliography.   4. Sex behavior—
Drug effects—Bibliography.   ZQV 84 A139a]
    Z6671.2.F46A26   [RG629.F45]   016.6183   82-6202
ISBN 0-313-23474-4   (lib. bdg.)   AACR2

Library of Congress Catalog Card Number: 82-6202
ISBN: 0-313-23474-4

First published in 1982

Greenwood Press
A division of Congressional Information Service, Inc.
88 Post Road West, Westport, Connecticut 06881

Printed in the United States of America

10 9 8 7 6 5 4 3 2 1

To my mother, Rose, who never stopped giving

Contents

Preface

This bibliography contains references to material dealing with alcohol's effects on reproduction. As such, it includes entries that deal with sexual behavior, sexual function, and sexual physiology, as well as alcohol's effects on the conceptus. The bulk of the entries, however, deal with "fetal alcohol syndrome." Some entries are listed "in press," since the terminal date for inclusion in this bibliography was 1981.

Although comprehensive, this bibliography is by no means exhaustive. Many of these entries were taken from my personal collection of materials. Entries were also collected from the reference lists included in these publications. Although many of the citations are not in English, I have translated these entries, or have used the translation provided in these materials. The title is presented in the original language, except in those instances where it was not possible to do so (for example, Japanese).

Entries are arranged alphabetically by author. A supplementary Addendum is also arranged in this way. These latter entries contain items that were inadvertently omitted in the initial listing or represent materials published after that listing. All items are numbered consecutively and are referred to by number in the Subject Index.

In compiling the Subject Index, I read many of the cited articles and based the indexing on the material included, rather than solely on the basis of title. This should provide a much more valuable guide to the literature than would be possible if titles alone were used.

In compiling a volume such as this, the services and cooperation of a great number of people are to be gratefully acknowledged. Among those who deserve special thanks are Charles Ernst, Dianne Augustino, and the librarians of the Health Sciences Library at the State University of New York at Buffalo.

Introduction

PHARMACOLOGY OF ALCOHOL

Alcohol (ethyl alcohol or ethanol [C_2H_5OH]) is a colorless, odorless liquid produced by fermentation. It is the main ingredient in all alcoholic beverages and is also found in various other materials such as medicines, lotions, and colognes.

Alcoholic beverages are divided into three main types: beers, wines, and distilled spirits. Beers contain about 3 to 6 percent alcohol; wines contain about 10 to 20 percent; and distilled spirits contain about 40 to 50 percent alcohol.

Beer is produced through the fermentation of grains such as corn, rye, barley, or wheat. Wines are produced through the fermentation of fruits such as the grape. Fermentation occurs when yeast converts the sugar in these substances into alcohol and carbon dioxide. In fermentation only about 14 percent of the final product contains alcohol. Wines with a higher alcohol content are "fortified" by adding additional alcohol.

Distilled spirits such as whiskey and bourbon are produced by heating fermented alcohol in a still. The alcohol boils off as vapor and is then recaptured and cooled, forming a much more concentrated solution of alcohol. Distilled spirits or liquors are frequently rated in terms of "proof." Proof is an archaic term referring to twice the percentage of alcohol in a beverage. One hundred proof is thus 50 percent alcohol. Various ingredients such as aldehydes and acids, or other forms of alcohol such as methyl or butyl alcohol may also be formed in the distillation process, or may be added in some form to give flavor to the beverage. These other ingredients are termed congeners.

Alcohol is readily absorbed from the small intestine into the blood and is distributed throughout the body. The rate of absorption varies according to the amount of food in the stomach (food delays absorption), the rate at which the alcohol is ingested (the faster it is drunk, the more alcohol in the blood), the concentration of the alcoholic beverage (the higher the concentration, the faster the rate of absorption), and the amount of alcohol consumed. The concentration in the blood is also affected by body weight (the heavier person has more blood in which the alcohol can distribute itself)and rate of metabolism (the rate at which alcohol is removed from the blood and broken down).

The reaction to alcohol is determined more as a result of its concentration in the blood than by the actual amount consumed. It is for this reason that two people may consume the same amount of alcohol and not be affected to the same extent. For example, if a 200 pound person and a 100 pound person consumed equal amounts of alcohol, the smaller individual would probably be affected to a greater degree, all other factors being equal. The volume of distribution would be less, resulting in a greater concentration of alcohol in the blood.

The concentration of alcohol in the blood is referred to usually as gram percent or milligram percent. This is the weight of alcohol in 100 milliliters of blood. A blood alcohol concentration (BAC) of 0.1 percent would be 0.1 grams of alcohol in 100 milliliters of blood (gram percent) or 100 milligrams of alcohol in 100 milliliters of blood (milligram percent).

After alcohol has entered the blood and is distributed to the liver, it begins to undergo a breakdown process called metabolism. Alcohol is initially broken down into acetaldehyde, a rather toxic substance. Usually little acetaldehyde accumulates in the blood because it is rapidly metabolized into acetate, which is then broken down into various other substances. The final breakdown products are water and carbon dioxide. About 95 percent of the alcohol taken into the body is metabolized. The remaining 5 percent is given off through the breath, perspiration, and urine.

In the adult human the rate of alcohol elimination from the body is about 0.015 percent per hour. This rate is about three to five times slower than in laboratory animals such as the mouse and the rat. The rate of elimination in the newborn infant is about 50 percent that of the adult. Elimination of alcohol from the fetus occurs primarily as a result of passive diffusion back across the placenta. The elimination of alcohol from the fetus thus depends on the rate of elimination of the mother.

As in the case of other tissues in the body, alcohol readily crosses the placenta and enters the fetus. The concentration of alcohol in the fetus is about the same as that in the mother. It is for this reason that some prevention campaigns point out that "a pregnant women never drinks alone."

PREVALENCE OF ALCOHOL CONSUMPTION

Compared to other countries the United States ranks fifteenth in overall consumption of alcohol, with an estimated intake of 2.7 gallons of absolute alcohol (100 percent) per adult annually. However, this estimate is misleading because it is based on the total adult population and includes both drinkers and nondrinkers. If alcohol consumption is based only on the 100 million adults who drink, then the estimated annual consumption is about 3.9 gallons of absolute alcohol. Expressed as "drinks" this converts into about 1,000 cans of beer or glasses of wine or distilled spirits or combination thereof.

This estimate is also misleading, since it does not take into account individual differences in consumption. One means of doing so has involved breaking down total consumption into categories such as "light," "moderate," and "heavy" drinkers. The criteria and estimated prevalence for each of these categories is as follows: "Light" drinking involves consumption of up to 0.5 drinks per day, 3 drinks per week, or 12 drinks per month (about 52 million Americans); "moderate" drinking involves consumption of between 4 and 13 drinks per week or 13 to 58 drinks per month (about 32 million Americans); and "heavy" drinking involves consumption of 2 or more drinks per day or 14 or more drinks per week (about 16 million Americans).

EFFECTS ON SEXUAL BEHAVIOR, FUNCTION, AND PHYSIOLOGY

Alcohol has been considered in the class of aphrodisiacs for centuries. For example, in the twelfth century, Maimonides wrote that "drinking honey water promotes erections, but ever more effective in this regard than all medicines and food is wine. . . ."

A sixteenth-century German writer extolled beer for similar reasons, stating that "beer brewed from wheat, above all as a beverage. . . increases the natural seed, straightens the drooping phallus up again, and helps feeble men who are incapable of conjugal acts back into the saddle."

Possibly the most frequently quoted statement on alcohol's effects regarding sex is in Shakespeare's Macbeth (Act 2, scene 2): "It (alcohol) provokes and unprovokes: it provokes the desire, but it takes away from the performance."

Although there is no shortage of anecdotal information concerning alcohol's relation to sex, there is by contrast very little in the way of carefully controlled studies of this relationship. Moreover, most of the available information concerns men. Very little has been done to investigate how alcohol affects female sexuality.

One of the more consistent findings with respect to alcohol and sexual function in men is that chronic alcoholism often results in impotence. In one study involving over 17,000 male alcoholics, about 8 percent were found to be impotent. Even after years of sobriety, about one-half of this number remained impotent, even though they still expressed a strong desire for sex. Another study reported a 31 percent incidence of erectile impotence and an 18 percent incidence of ejaculatory failure among a group of forty-five male alcoholics.

Controlled laboratory studies have corroborated these findings. Using college students and a penile strain gauge to measure tumescence, researchers have observed a dose-related inhibition in penile tumescence associated with ingestion of alcohol.

Studies on paraplegic animals and men suggest that one of the ways alcohol causes impotence is by affecting the spinal reflex centers underlying erectile and ejaculatory processes. For example, in one study subarachnoid injection of alcohol was observed to inhibit priapism in paraplegic men. In another study, erectile and ejaculatory reflexes in dogs with mid-thoracic spinal transections were abolished by alcohol.

Although studies such as these indicate that alcohol can directly inhibit spinal neural mechanisms underlying tumescence and ejaculation, this does not preclude alcohol's affecting similar functions mediated by higher cortical centers or through hormonal mechanisms.

The relationship between alcohol consumption and hormonal mechanisms relating to sexual physiology has been, in fact, actively studied in contrast to alcohol's effects on sexual behavior. In general, these studies have shown that chronic alcohol consumption often leads to feminization in men—for example, hypogonadism, gynecomastia, and decreased beard and pubic hair. Although such feminization may be the result of alcohol related liver dysfunction, recent studies have shown that such changes can also occur independent of alcohol's effects on the liver.

A frequent observation among alcoholics and in animals chronically treated with alcohol is a decrease in serum testosterone levels. Clinical and experimental studies suggest that this decrease arises through a dual action of alcohol. On the one hand, alcohol appears to cause damage to the Leydig cells in the testes which are involved in the production of testosterone, and on the other, it appears to inhibit the hypothalamic-pituitary-gonadal axis by which the pituitary influences the testes to produce testosterone.

In terms of reproduction per se, one of the most important effects of chronic ingestion of alcohol is sperm damage. Alcohol not only inhibits sperm motility but also causes changes in sperm itself such as curled tails, distended midsections, and broken heads. Sterility may also occur as a direct result of alcohol's actions on gonadal tissues, or by causing obstruction of the vas deferens.

With respect to female sexuality, self-report studies of sexual attitudes and behavior suggest that female alcoholics are more likely to desire and engage in intercourse than nonalcoholics. A laboratory study using the vaginal photoplethysmograph, an instrument to measure vaginal pressure, indicated that alcohol causes a dose-related decrease in vaginal pressure, but at the same time the women in this study stated that they felt more sexually aroused with increasing blood alcohol levels.

Chronic alcohol ingestion in women, as in men, results in various adverse effects on reproductive physiology. Among the obstetrical gynecological problems related to alcohol consumption are menstrual disorders, miscarriage, infertility, and difficulties in labor. Studies of animals have shown that chronic ingestion of alcohol can result in atrophy of the ovary, uterus, and fallopian tubes.

FETAL ALCOHOL SYNDROME

Concern over the potential harmful effects of alcohol on the developing fetus can be traced back to the time of the Greeks. Plato, for example cautioned that "it is not right that procreation should be the work of bodies dissolved by excess wine, but rather that the embryo should be compacted firmly, steadily, and quietly in the womb."

Aristotle likewise observed that "foolish, drunken, or hare-brained women (for the) most part bring forth children like unto themselves, morose and languid."

Although these warnings and observations have been noted several times hence, most notably during the so-called "gin epidemic" of the eighteenth century in England, it was not until the publication in 1973 in *Lancet* by two physicians, K. L. Jones and D. W. Smith, that worldwide attention was focused on a pattern of alcohol-related birth defects, which has come to be known as fetal alcohol syndrome.

The primary features of this syndrome are prenatal and postnatal growth retardation, especially microcephaly (small head); facial anomalies such as indistinctive philtrum (the groove between the nose and mouth), and low-set unparallel ears; limb, joint, and organ disorders that often involve the heart and kidney; and behavioral or cognitive impairment such as subnormal intelligence, fine motor dysfunction, and hyperactivity. Although growth retardation and physical anomalies are the most visible aspects of this syndrome, the cognitive impairments are the most serious characteristics. In fact, maternal alcohol abuse during pregnancy is regarded as one of the most common teratogenic causes of mental deficiency in the Western world.

Although the actual number of children born with fetal alcohol syndrome is unknown, estimates place the number at one to two live births per 1,000 normal births. Instances of the syndrome have now been observed in Australia, Belgium, Brazil, Canada, Chile, Czechoslovakia, France, Germany, Hungary, Ireland, Italy, Japan, Reunion, Scotland, South Africa, Spain, Sweden, Switzerland, and the United States. The syndrome is thus ubiquitous and not confined to any one country or any particular part of the world.

Although much interest has been focused on fetal alcohol syndrome as a clinical entity, *in utero* alcohol exposure is associated with adverse effects ranging from spontaneous abortion and perinatal death at one extreme to neurological disorders in the absence of visible physical anomalies at the other. The overall incidence of these "fetal alcohol effects" is estimated at three to five live births per 1,000 (not including spontaneous abortions). A partial list of fetal alcohol effects is presented in Table 1.

Table 1
Effects Associated with Prenatal Exposure to Alcohol

Growth
intrauterine growth retardation
postnatal growth retardation
microcephaly

Facial
short palpebral fissures
indistinct philtrum
epicanthic folds
strabismus
ptosis
shortened upturned nasal bridge
antimongoloid fissures
thin lips
underdeveloped jaw
high arched palate
low set ears
posteriorly rotated ears
cleft palate
anomalies of the teeth
midface hypoplasia

Limb/Joint Skeletal Anomalies
abnormal palmar creases
clinodactyly
campodactyly
hypoplasia of nails
hip dislocation

Chest
funnel breast

General
hirsutism

Cardiovascular Defects
atrial septal defect
ventricular septal defect
pulmonary stenosis
ductus arteriosus

Kidney Anomalies
hydronephrosis
renal hypoplasia
agenesis of kidney

Neural Tube Defects
anencephaly
myelomeningomyelocele
sacral meningomyelocele
lumbar meningomyelocele

Neuropathological Defects
incomplete cortical development
enlarged ventricles
fusion of ventricles
aberrant neuronal and and glial
  migration
absence or underdevelopment of corpus
  callosum
absence of anterior commisure
rudimentary cerebellum
absence of olfactory bulbs

Behavioral Anomalies
mental retardation
hyperactivity
sleep disorders
irritability
psychomotor defects

In general, the degree of behavioral impairment tends to be positively correlated with the degree of physical anomalies, but behavioral impairment may occur in conjunction with only minor or no observable physical defects. In such instances it may be very difficult to determine alcohol's behavioral teratogenicity. For this reason many researchers have devoted considerable effort to investigating the prenatal effects of alcohol in animals. Among the many advantages of such experimentation is the shorter lifespan of an "animal model," which enables a better assessment of the link between *in utero* alcohol exposure and adult behavioral impairment.

Studies in animals have demonstrated that alcohol is unquestionably a teratogen. These studies have also demonstrated that alcohol does not produce its teratogenic actions through secondary mechanisms such as maternal undernutrition. Although alcohol contains about seven calories per gram and can partially satisfy daily caloric requirements so that less food is eaten, studies in animals using the "pair-feeding" technique have been able to control for this potentially confounding factor in assessing alcohol's actions on the developing fetus. The essence of this technique involves establishing two groups of animals. One group is given alcohol and is permitted unlimited access to food. The second "control" group is given an isocaloric substance and is only permitted an amount of food equal to that consumed by the animals in the alcohol treated group. By comparing the two groups, which differ only in terms of alcohol administration, researchers are able to assess the role of alcohol independently of its nutritional effects as far as maternal food consumption is concerned.

Studies in animals have also enabled researchers to rule out the contribution of other factors generally associated with alcohol consumption in humans such as smoking. In many cases women who drink heavily also smoke heavily, and it is difficult to differentiate between alcohol's effects and the effects of smoking. Smoking, for example, also results in lower birth weight. Animal experimentation resolves this problem by enabling researchers to control the life histories so that alcohol can be studied in and of itself, rather than in conjunction with smoking. In addition, researchers can also administer tobacco products to animals to determine if there are any interactive effects. These studies also eliminate other factors associated with heavy drinking as primary mechanisms responsible for alcohol's influence on the developing fetus, such as poor maternal health, poverty, and physical stress.

Much attention has been directed to determining what amount of drinking is dangerous to fetal development. This question is still unsettled and will probably remain so for some time yet. Because of the considerations concerning the absorption and metabolism of alcohol as noted above, there can be no general statement regarding "safe" levels of drinking. Moreover, in addition to pharmacological factors, there is also the consideration of possible genetic susceptibility. Studies in twins, for example, have shown that while both are exposed to the same amount of alcohol *in utero*, one twin may be more severely affected than another. Also to be considered is the physical condition of the mother herself. While nutritional factors may not be the primary cause of fetal alcohol effects, they may interact with alcohol exposure to produce such effects. Identifying risk factors, in addition to alcohol consumption, is important if clinicians are to best advise their patients concerning drinking.

Exposure during development when alcohol would be most damaging is another area of interest. Although the conceptus is most vulnerable to gross anatomical malformations during the period of organogenesis (the first twelve weeks in humans, the first two weeks in rodents), insults to development may still occur after this period. The so-called "critical period" for growth retardation has been found to be the latter third of pregnancy in humans and animals. Recent studies also suggest that this may also be a sensitive period for insult to brain development, which can result in behavioral anomalies.

One means by which alcohol appears to affect development is by inhibiting protein synthesis in the developing fetus. This may occur through inhibition of placental transport of amino acids, or through inhibition of the biological mechanisms responsible for incorporation of these amino acids into protein. Since accumulation of protein is essential for increased cellular growth and proliferation, such inhibition is not an improbable cause of the growth retardation associated with in utero alcohol exposure. Inhibition of protein synthesis can also result in malformations if essential "building blocks" are unavailable.

Alcohol may affect protein synthesis and other developmental processes by causing fetal hypoxia. Growth retardation and various behavioral anomalies such as mental retardation and hyperactivity may be caused by fetal hypoxia, and it could also be a factor in damage to developing organs. Alcohol has been shown to inhibit incorporation of amino acids into proteins, and this could be the basis for some of the effects associated with in utero alcohol exposure.

There is considerable evidence to indicate that alcohol causes fetal hypoxia. Cessation of breathing movements of the fetus for longer than fifty minutes has been observed after women consumed about one ounce of vodka. Decreased fetal respiration has also been reported in studies in which alcohol was used as an anesthetic during pregnancy. In a study assessing neonatal outcome in infants born to women who received alcohol to prevent premature labor, those infants born within twelve hours of alcohol exposure had a considerably higher than normal incidence of respiratory problems.

Animal studies also indicate possible fetal hypoxia from in utero alcohol exposure. In fetal sheep, for example, blood oxygen content was significantly reduced following maternal alcohol infusion. When alcohol was administered to pregnant monkeys, feteral arterial blood pressure decreased and acidity of the blood and heart rate increased—changes that were interpreted as evidence of fetal hypoxia.

Women who drink heavily also have a higher incidence of pregnancy complications associated with fetal hypoxia than do other women, for example, placenta praevia, antepartum bleeding, and anemia. Infants born to alcoholic women also have a higher incidence of meconium staining, a generally accepted indicant of fetal hypoxia.

Some researchers have argued that the critical factor in determining whether or not a woman will give birth to a child with fetal alcohol syndrome is the blood acetaldehyde levels occurring in her blood. This hypothesis contends that due to peculiarities in the way the liver metabolizes alcohol and/or acetaldehyde, toxic levels of acetaldehyde build up in the blood and are transferred to the fetus. Against this hypothesis, however, are those demonstrations of decreased growth in embryos that are exposed to alcohol *in vitro*, where there is minimal conversion of alcohol to acetaldehyde.

There are two other considerations that have generated some attention with respect to fetal alcohol syndrome. The first is the possible contribution of paternal factors. As noted previously, many male alcoholics are impotent or sterile, and those that are not may produce sperm that are abnormal. If these sperm are able to fertilize an ovum, there is the possibility of an abnormal offspring being born. This possibility has received some support in a number of animal studies wherein males chronically treated with alcohol were allowed to breed with females that were not exposed to alcohol.

The second consideration is that alcohol may somehow have lasting effects on female reproductive mechanisms, which place a woman at-risk for fetal alcohol effects. Such a suggestion is supported by studies of recovered alcoholics who did not drink during pregnancy but whose children still differed in birth weight from those born to nonalcoholics.

Despite the fact that much more remains to be discovered regarding alcohol's effects on the developing fetus, several prevention/education programs have already been initiated to alert obstericians and the public to the potential risks of drinking during pregnancy. These programs have been carried out at both local and state levels. In some cases these programs advise abstinence during pregnancy, whereas in others no such advice is given. A recent opinion survey indicated that nearly all women of childbearing age (92 percent) have been made aware of the possibility of birth defects arising out of drinking during pregnancy, which is probably due to the efforts of these programs.

Bibliography

1. AASE, J. (1980) 'FAS in American Indians: A high risk group.'
    Paper presented at the Fetal Alcohol Syndrome Workshop, Seat-
    tle, Washington (May 2-4).

2. AASE, J. (1981) 'The fetal alcohol syndrome in American Indians:
    A high risk group.' Neurobehavioral Toxicology and Tera-
    tology, 3, 153-156.

3. AASLAND, T. (1979) 'Det føtale alkoholsyndrom: Fosterskadene
    langt alvorliegere enn tidligere antatt.' ['The fetal alco-
    hol syndrome: Damage of the fetus more serious than antici-
    pated.'] Tidsskrift om Edruskaps Spørsmal, 31, 3, 15.

4. ABEL, E.L. (1974) 'Alcohol ingestion in lactating rats: Effects
    on mothers and offspring. I.' Archives Internationales de
    Pharmacodynamie et de Thérapie (Gand), 210, 121-126.

5. ABEL, E.L. (1975) 'Emotionality in offspring of rats fed alcohol
    while nursing.' Journal of Studies on Alcohol, 36, 654-658.

6. ABEL, E.L. (1978) 'Effects of ethanol on pregnant rats and
    their offspring.' Psychopharmacology (Berlin), 57, 5-11.

7. ABEL, E.L. (1979) 'Effects of alcohol withdrawal and under-
    nutrition on cannibalism of rat pups.' Behavioral and
    Neural Biology, 25, 411-413.

8. ABEL, E.L. (1979) 'Effects of ethanol exposure during different
    gestation weeks of pregnancy on maternal weight gain and
    intrauterine growth retardation in the rat.' Neurobehav-
    ioral Toxicology, 1, 145-151.

9. ABEL, E.L. (1979) 'Effects of lactation on rate of blood ethanol
    disappearance, ethanol consumption and serum electrolytes in
    the rat.' Bulletin of the Psychonomic Society, 14, 365-367.

10. ABEL, E.L. (1979) 'Prenatal effects of alcohol on adult learning
    in rats.' Pharmacology, Biochemistry, and Behavior, 10,
    239-243.

11. ABEL, E.L. (1979) 'Prenatal effects of alcohol on open-field behavior, step-down latencies and "sleep time."' Behavioral and Neural Biology, 25, 406-410.

12. ABEL, E.L. (1979) 'Sex ratio in fetal alcohol syndrome.' Lancet (London), 2, 105.

13. ABEL, E.L. (1980) 'A review of alcohol's effects on sex and reproduction.' Drug and Alcohol Dependence, 5, 321-332.

14. ABEL, E.L. (1980) 'Effects of beverage alcohols on growth.' Paper presented at the Fetal Alcohol Syndrome Workshop, Seattle, Washington (May 2-4).

15. ABEL, E.L. (1980) 'Prenatal exposure to ethanol or alcoholic beverages: Effects on postnatal body weight and food and water consumption.' Paper presented at the International Society for Developmental Psychobiology, Cincinnati (November 8).

16. ABEL, E.L. (1980) Presentation of testimony at public hearings on the New York State Five-Year Plan for the Division of Alcoholism and Alcohol Abuse, Buffalo, New York (November 21).

17. ABEL, E.L. (1980) 'Procedural considerations in evaluating prenatal effects of alcohol in animals.' Teratology, 21, 25A (abstract).

18. ABEL, E.L. (1980) 'Procedural considerations in evaluating prenatal effects of alcohol in animals.' Neurobehavioral Toxicology, 2, 167-174.

19. ABEL, E.L. (1980) 'The fetal alcohol syndrome: Behavioral teratology.' Psychological Bulletin, 87, 29-50.

20. ABEL, E.L. (1981) 'A critical evaluation of the obstetric use of alcohol in preterm labor.' Drug and Alcohol Dependence, 7, 367-378.

21. ABEL, E.L. (1981) 'Behavioral teratology of alcohol.' Psychological Bulletin , 90, 564-581.

22. ABEL, E.L. (1981) 'Behavioral teratology of alcohol.' In: Fetal Alcohol Syndrome. Volume 3: Animal Studies. Ed. E.L. Abel. Boca Raton, Florida: CRC Press (in press).

23. ABEL, E.L. (1981) 'Consumption of alcohol during pregnancy: Effects on growth and development of offspring.' Human Biology (in press).

24. ABEL, E.L. (1981) Fetal Alcohol Syndrome. Volume 1: An Annotated and Comprehensive Bibliography. Boca Raton, Florida: CRC Press.

25. ABEL, E.L. (1981) Fetal Alcohol Syndrome. Volume 2: Human
         Studies. Boca Raton, Florida: CRC Press.

26. ABEL, E.L. (1981) Fetal Alcohol Syndrome. Volume 3: Animal
         Studies. Boca Raton, Florida: CRC Press.

27. ABEL, E.L. (1981) 'Prenatal alcohol exposure affects adult
         responsiveness to drugs.' Alcoholism: Clinical and Exper-
         imental Research, 5, 142 (abstract).

28. ABEL, E.L. (1981) 'Prenatal effects of beverage alcohol on fetal
         growth.' Progress in Biochemical Pharmacology, 18, 111.

29. ABEL, E.L. (1981) 'Prenatal exposure to beer, wine, whiskey, or
         ethanol: Effects on fetal body weight in rats.' Paper pre-
         sented at the Annual Meeting of the American Association for
         the Advancement of Science, Toronto, Canada (January).

30. ABEL, E.L. (1981) 'Prenatal exposure to beer, wine, whiskey,
         and ethanol: Effects on postnatal growth and food and water
         consumption.' Neurobehavioral Toxicology and Teratology, 3,
         49-51.

31. ABEL, E.L., BUSH, R., and DINTCHEFF, B.A. (1981) 'Exposure of
         rats to alcohol in utero alters drug sensitivity in adult-
         hood.' Science, 212, 1531-1533.

32. ABEL, E.L., and DINTCHEFF, B.A. (1978) 'Effects of prenatal
         alcohol exposure on growth and development in rats.' Jour-
         nal of Pharmacology and Experimental Therapeutics, 207,
         916-921.

33. ABEL, E.L., DINTCHEFF, B.A., and BUSH, R. (1981) 'Behavioral
         teratology of alcoholic beverages compared to ethanol.'
         Neurobehavioral Toxicology and Teratology, 3, 339-342.

34. ABEL, E.L., DINTCHEFF, B.A., and BUSH, R. (1981) 'Effects of
         beer, wine, whiskey, and ethanol on pregnant rats and their
         offspring.' Teratology, 23, 217-222.

35. ABEL, E.L., DINTCHEFF, B.A., and DAY, N. (1979) 'Effects of in
         utero exposure to alcohol, nicotine, and alcohol plus nico-
         tine, on growth and development in rats.' Neurobehavioral
         Toxicology, 1, 153-159.

36. ABEL, E.L., and GREIZERSTEIN, H.B. (1979) 'Ethanol-induced pre-
         natal growth deficiency: Changes in fetal body composition.'
         Journal of Pharmacology and Experimental Therapeutics, 211,
         668-671.

37. ABEL, E.L., and GREIZERSTEIN, H.B. (1979) 'In utero exposure to
         ethanol: Effects on fetal development in rats.' Pharma-
         ologist, 21, 222 (Abstract #413).

38. ABEL, E.L., and GREIZERSTEIN, H.B. (1980) 'Relation of alcohol content in amniotic fluid, fetal and maternal blood.' Alcoholism: Clinical and Experimental Research, 4, 209 (abstract).

39. ABEL, E.L., and GREIZERSTEIN, H.B. (1981) 'Growth and development in animals prenatally exposed to alcohol.' In: Fetal Alcohol Syndrome. Volume 3: Animal Studies. Ed. E.L. Abel. Boca Raton, Florida: CRC Press (in press).

40. ABEL, E.L., GREIZERSTEIN, H.B., and SIEMENS, A.J. (1979) 'Influence of lactation on rate of disappearance of ethanol in the rat.' Neurobehavioral Toxicology, 1, 185-196.

41. ABEL, E.L., RANDALL, C.L., and RILEY, E.P. (1981) 'Alcohol consumption and prenatal development.' In: Medical and Social Aspects of Alcohol Abuse. Ed. B. Tabikoff, P.B. Sutker, and C.L. Randall. New York: Plenum Press (in press).

42. ABEL, E.L., and YORK, J.L. (1979) 'Absence of effect of prenatal ethanol on adult emotionality and ethanol consumption in rats.' Journal of Studies on Alcohol, 40, 547-553.

43. ABRAMOWITZ, J., and BIRNBAUMER, L. (1979) 'Effects of trypsin, protease inhibitors and ethanol on corpus luteum adenyl cyclase.' Biology of Reproduction, 21, 213-217.

44. ADAM, F., and GENSOLLEN, G. (1914) 'Contribution à l'étude de l'alcoolisme chronique chez les enfants.' ['Contribution to the study of chronic alcoholism in infants.'] Enfance Abnormale, 3, 276-278.

45. ADAMS, J. (1979) 'Behavioral assessment of the teratogenous effects of prenatal exposure to ethanol in the rat.' Teratology, 19, 17A (abstract).

46. AKESSON, C. (1974) 'Autoradiographic studies on the distribution of ^{14}C-2-ethanol and its non-volatile metabolites in the pregnant mouse.' Archives Internationales de Pharmacodynamie et de Thérapie (Gand), 209, 296-304.

47. AKHTAR, M.J. (1977) 'Sexual disorders in male alcoholics.' In: Alcoholism and Drug Dependence: A Multidisciplinary Approach. Ed. J.S. Madden, R. Walker, and W.H. Kenyon. New York: Plenum Press, pp. 3-12.

48. ALPERT, J.J. (1980) 'The Boston study.' Paper presented at the Fetal Alcohol Syndrome Workshop, Seattle, Washington (May 2-4).

49. ALPERT, J.J., DAY, N., DOOLING, E., HINGSON, R., OPPENHEIMER, E., ROSETT, H.L., WEINER, L., and ZUCKERMAN, B. (1981) 'Maternal alcohol consumption and new-born assessment: Methodology of the Boston City Hospital prospective study.' Neurobehavioral Toxicology and Teratology, 3, 195-201.

50. ALTMAN, B.   (1976) 'Fetal alcohol syndrome.' Journal of Ped-
        iatric Ophthalmology, 13, 255-258.

51. ALTMAN, G.B. (1980) 'Prevention of the effects of alcohol on the
        unborn baby by the development of education programs.' Paper
        presented at the National Council on Alcoholism Conference,
        Seattle, Washington (May 2-4).

52. ALTSHULER, G., PEARSON, R., ALTMILLER, D., and KUHN, J. (1980)
        'The fetal alcohol syndrome: Considerations of acute and
        chronic rat models.' Laboratory Investigations, 42, 98 (ab-
        stract).

53. ALTSHULER, H.L. (1980) 'A subhuman primate model of FAS.' Paper
        presented at the Fetal Alcohol Syndrome Workshop, Seattle,
        Washington (May 2-4).

54. ALTSHULER, H.L., and SHIPPENBERG, T.S. (1981) 'A subhuman prim-
        ate model for fetal alcohol syndrome research.' Neurobehav-
        ioral Toxicology and Teratology, 3, 121-126.

55. ALVAREZ, M.R., CIMINO, L.E., JR., CORY, M.J., and GORDON, R.E.
        (1980) 'Ethanol induction of sister chromatid exchanges in
        human cells in vitro.' Cytogenetic Cell Genetics, 27, 66-69.

56. ALVAREZ, M.R., CIMINO, L.E., JR., and PUSATERI, T.J. (1980) 'In-
        duction of sister chromatid exchanges in mouse fetuses re-
        sulting from maternal alcohol consumption during pregnancy.'
        Cytogenetic Cell Genetics, 28, 173-180.

57. ANANDAM, N., FELEGI, W., and STERN, J. (1979) 'Fetal alcohol en-
        hances auditory startle in rats.' Paper presented at the In-
        ternational Society for Developmental Psychobiology, Atlanta,
        Georgia (November).

58. ANANDAM, N., FELEGI, W., and STERN, J. (1980) 'In utero alcohol
        heightens juvenile reactivity.' Pharmacology, Biochemistry,
        and Behavior, 13, 531-535.

59. ANANDAM, N.T., and STERN, J.M. (1980) 'Alcohol in utero: Ef-
        fects on preweanling appetitive learning.' Neurobehavioral
        Toxicology, 2, 199-205.

60. ANANDAM, N.T., STRAIT, T., and STERN, J.M. (1980) 'In utero
        ethanol retards early discrimination learning and decreases
        adult responsiveness to ethanol.' Teratology, 21, 25A (ab-
        stract).

61. ANDERS, K., and PERSAUD, T.V.N. (1981) 'Compensatory embryonic
      / development in the rat following maternal treatment with
        ethanol.' Anatomical Record, 199, 144 (abstract).

62. ANDERSON, C.M. (1972) 'Minimal brain damage.' Mental Hygiene,
        56, 62-66.

63. ANDERSON, D.C. (1978) 'The effect of alcohol on the hepatic
        metabolism of hormones.' European Journal of Clinical
        Investigation (Berlin), 8, 267-268.

64. ANDERSON, R.A., JR. (1980) 'Effects of male alcoholism.' Paper
        presented at the Fetal Alcohol Syndrome Workshop, Seattle,
        Washington (May 2-4).

65. ANDERSON, R.A., JR. (1980) 'Ethanol effects on hormonal milieu
        and fetal development.' Paper presented at the Fetal Alco-
        hol Syndrome Workshop, Seattle, Washington (May 2-4).

66. ANDERSON, R.A., JR. (1981) 'Endocrine balance as a factor in the
        etiology of the fetal alcohol syndrome.' Neurobehavioral
        Toxicology and Teratology, 3, 89-104.

67. ANDERSON, R.A., JR. (1981) 'The possible role of paternal alco-
        hol consumption in the etiology of the fetal alcohol syn-
        drome.' In: Fetal Alcohol Syndrome. Volume 2: Human
        Studies. Ed. E.L. Abel. Boca Raton, Florida: CRC Press
        (in press).

68. ANDERSON, R.A., JR., and BEYLER, S.A. (1978) 'Reduced litter
        size and survival of offspring sired by ethanol treated male
        mice.' Biology of Reproduction, 18 (Supplement 1), 49a
        (abstract).

69. ANDERSON, R.A., JR., BEYLER, S.A., and ZANEVELD, L.J.D. (1978)
        'Alterations of male reproduction induced by chronic inges-
        tion of ethanol: Development of an animal model.' Fertility
        and Sterility, 30, 103-105.

70. ANDERSON, R.A., JR., FURBY, J.E., OSWALD, C., and ZANEVELD, L.Z.D.
        (1981) 'Teratological evaluation of mouse fetuses after
        paternal alcohol ingestion.' Neurobehavioral Toxicology and
        Teratology, 3, 117-120.

71. ANDERSON, R.A., JR., REDDY, J.M., OSWALD, C., WILLIS, B., and
        ZANEVELD, L.J.D. (1980) 'Decreased male fertility induced
        by chronic alcohol ingestion.' Federation Proceedings, 39,
        541 (abstract).

72. ANDERSON, R.A., JR., WILLIS, B.R., OSWALD, C., GUPTA, A., and
        ZANEVELD, L.J.D. (1981) 'Delayed male sexual maturation
        induced by chronic ethanol ingestion.' Federation Pro-
        ceedings, 40, 825 (abstract).

73. ANDERSON, R.A., JR., WILLIS, B.R., OSWALD, C., REDDY, J.M., BEY-
        LER, S.A., and ZANEVELD, L.J.D. (1980) 'Hormonal imbalance
        and alterations in testicular morphology induced by chronic
        ingestion of ethanol.' Biochemical Pharmacology, 29, 1409-
        1419.

74. ANDERSON, W. (1979) 'A study of brain alterations in postnatal
        rats induced by alcohol intoxication.' Anatomical Record,
        193, 471 (abstract).

75. ANDERSON, W.J., and SIDES, G.R. (1979) 'Alcohol induced defects
        in cerebellar development in the rat.' In: Currents in
        Alcoholism. Volume 5: Biomedical Issues and Clinical Ef-
        fects of Alcoholism. Ed. Marc Galanter. New York: Grune
        and Stratton, pp. 135-153.

76. ANONYMOUS. (1907) 'Welcher Einfluss hat der Alkoholismus eines
        oder beider Eltern auf die Nachkommenschaft?' ['What influ-
        ence has the alcoholism of one or both parents on the off-
        spring?'] Zeitschrift für Socialwissenschaft, 4, 250.

77. ANONYMOUS. (1942) 'Effect of single large alcohol intake on
        fetus.' (Queries and Minor Notes.) Journal of the American
        Medical Association, 120, 88.

78. ANONYMOUS. (1947) 'Alcohol, heredity and germ damage.' Quarter-
        ly Journal of Studies on Alcohol (Supplement), No. 5, n. pag.

79. ANONYMOUS. (1949) 'Effect of alcohol and tobacco on fertility.'
        (Any Questions?) British Medical Journal (London), 2, 768.

80. ANONYMOUS. (1954) 'Smoking and drinking during pregnancy.'
        (Queries and Minor Notes.) Journal of the American Medical
        Association, 154, 186.

81. ANONYMOUS. (1955) 'Chronic alcoholism and fertility.' (Any
        Questions?) British Medical Journal (London), 1, 1170.

82. ANONYMOUS. (1971) 'Alcoholic mothers' babies fail to thrive.'
        Journal of the American Medical Association, 213, 1429-1450.

83. ANONYMOUS. (1974) 'Alcoholism and women.' Alcohol Health and
        Research World, Experimental Issue, pp. 2-7.

84. ANONYMOUS. (1974) 'Children of alcoholic mothers fail to thrive
        physically and mentally.' Journal of the American Medical
        Association, 229, 9.

85. ANONYMOUS. (1975) 'À propos de la descendance des alcooliques.'
        ['Concerning the offspring of alcoholics.'] Revue de l'Al-
        coolisme (Paris), 21, xvii-xviii.

86. ANONYMOUS. (1975) '"Bottle" babies.' Listen, May.

87. ANONYMOUS. (1975) 'Libido of female alcoholics.' (Questions and
        Answers.) Medical Aspects of Human Sexuality, 9, 99.

88. ANONYMOUS. (1975) "Pediatricians finding fetal alcohol effects.'
        U.S. Medicine, p. 15.

89. ANONYMOUS. (1975) 'Study shows rise in drunk newborns.' Jet
        Magazine, May 29.

90. ANONYMOUS. (1976) 'Fetal alcohol syndrome.' [Editorial.]
        British Medical Journal (London), 2, 1404-1405.

91. ANONYMOUS. (1976) 'Fetal alcohol syndrome.' [Editorial.] Lan-
       cet (London), 1, 1335.

92. ANONYMOUS. (1976) 'Heart defects accompany fetal alcohol syn-
       drome.' (Medical News.) Journal of the American Medical
       Association, 235, 2073.

93. ANONYMOUS. (1977) 'Can alcoholic fathers cause birth defects?'
       Listen, 3-4.

94. ANONYMOUS. (1977) 'Da hilft nur Verzicht auf Alkohol und Zigar-
       etten: Schwangere Gefährden ihr King-Wissenschaftliche
       Studie über "Schwangerschaftsverlauf und Kindesentwicklung."'
       ['So only renunciation of alcohol and cigarettes helps:
       Pregnancy risks to her in King's scientific study on "Course
       of pregnancy and child development."'] Schwestern Revue, 15,
       11-12.

95. ANONYMOUS. (1977) 'Even moderate drinking may be hazardous to
       maturing fetus.' (Medical News.) Journal of the American
       Medical Association, 237, 2585-2587.

96. ANONYMOUS. (1977) 'Fetal alcohol syndrome.' FDA Drug Bulletin,
       7, 18.

97. ANONYMOUS. (1977) 'Pregnancy in the heavy drinker.' Lancet
       (London), 2, 647.

98. ANONYMOUS. (1977) 'The fetal alcohol syndrome: A threat to our
       children.' The Globe, 2, 3.

99. ANONYMOUS. (1977) 'The fetal alcohol syndrome: Recent German
       investigations.' The Globe, 2, 5-7, 22.

100. ANONYMOUS. (1977) 'The spectre of fetal alcoholism.' Emergency
       Medicine, 9, 121-125.

101. ANONYMOUS. (1978) 'Can alcoholic fathers cause birth defects?'
       Listen, 3-4 (March).

102. ANONYMOUS. (1978) 'Effects of alcohol on the fetus.' [Letter.]
       New England Journal of Medicine, 298, 55-56.

103. ANONYMOUS. (1978) 'Fetal alcohol syndrome.' Current Health, 2,
       12-13.

104. ANONYMOUS. (1978) 'Fetal alcohol syndrome.' [Letter.] South
       African Medical Journal, 54, 552.

105. ANONYMOUS. (1978) 'Fetal alcohol syndrome: New perspectives.'
       Alcohol Health and Research World, 2, 2-12.

106. ANONYMOUS. (1978) 'Maternal alcohol consumption and birth
       weight.' British Medical Journal (London), 2, 76-77.

107. ANONYMOUS. (1978) 'Preventing the birth of a handicapped
          child?' Midwives Chronicle, 91, 34-36.

108. ANONYMOUS. (1978) 'Smoking, drinking, and pregnancy.' [Bro-
          chure.] Do It Now Foundation Institute for Chemical Sur-
          vival. Phoenix, Arizona.

109. ANONYMOUS. (1979) 'Alcohol level and offspring.' Science News,
          115, 41.

110. ANONYMOUS. (1979) 'Broad education program on drinking and preg-
          nancy.' Discus Newsletter, No. 384.

111. ANONYMOUS. (1979) 'Fetal alcohol syndrome.' [Editorial.] Pedi-
          atric Annals, 8, 119-120.

112. ANONYMOUS. (1979) 'March of Dimes joins educational effort.'
          Discus Newsletter, No. 386.

113. ANONYMOUS. (1979) 'Mother's ruin is baby's downfall.' New
          Scientist, 81, 76.

114. ANONYMOUS. (1979) 'Physicians sent advisory on drinking, preg-
          nancy.' Discus Newsletter, No. 386.

115. ANONYMOUS. (1979) 'Scientists study fetal alcohol syndrome.'
          Alcoholism Newsletter, 1, 1.

116. ANONYMOUS. (1979) 'Teratogenic activity of alcohol.' [In Ger-
          man.] Naturwissenschaftliche Rundschau, 32, 253-254.

117. ANONYMOUS. (1980) 'Abstinence or moderation for pregnant women?'
          The Globe, No. 2, 14-15.

118. ANONYMOUS. (1980) 'Alcohol and sex.' Bottom Line, 3, 17-18.

119. ANONYMOUS. (1980) 'Alcohol and spontaneous abortion.' [Editor-
          ial.] Lancet (London), 2, 188-189.

120. ANONYMOUS. (1980) 'Alcohol and your unborn baby.' AARN News
          Letter, 36, 1-2.

121. ANONYMOUS. (1980) 'Alcohol as a risk factor in pregnancy.'
          Unpublished report.

122. ANONYMOUS, (1980) 'Drinking doubles risk of birth abnormality.'
          Focus on Alcohol and Drug Issues, 3, 22.

123. ANONYMOUS. (1980) 'Perinatal and neonatal mortality: A welcome
          report.' [Leading articles.] British Medical Journal
          (London), 281, 255-256.

124. ANONYMOUS. (1980) 'The bad egg.' Lancet (London), 1, 690.

125. ANONYMOUS. (1980) 'The fetal alcohol syndrome--A threat to our
          children.' The Globe, No. 1, 14-15.

126. ANONYMOUS. (1980) 'The only sound advice: Women should not drink when pregnant.' The Globe, No. 4, 14.

127. ANONYMOUS. (1980) 'Warning--Alcohol may be hazardous to your baby.' American Pharmacy, 19, 688-689.

128. ANONYMOUS. (1981) 'ADAMHA has "great stake" in research on maternal, child health.' ADAMHA News (Alcohol, Drug Abuse, and Mental Health Administration), 7 (July 24), 1, 4, 6.

129. ANONYMOUS. (1981) 'Dr. Gomberg's view of FAS.' Discus Newsletter, No. 392.

130. ANONYMOUS. (1981) 'Dr. Rosett stresses need for medical training package.' Discus Newsletter, No. 393, p. 1, 4.

131. ANONYMOUS. (1981) 'Fetal alcohol syndrome.' Tijdschrift voor Ziekenverpleging, 34, 79.

132. ANONYMOUS. (1981) 'GPs leading pregnant women astray.' Medical News Weekly, 13 (October), 1.

133. ANONYMOUS. (1981) 'Moderate maternal drinking, birth anomalies unrelated.' Discus Newsletter, No. 393, p. 2.

134. ANONYMOUS (1981) 'Surgeon General's advisory on alcohol and pregnancy.' FDA Drug Bulletin, 11 (July), 1-2.

135. ANTON, G. (1901-1902) 'Alkoholismus und Erblichkeit.' ['Alcoholism and nausea.'] Psychologische Wochenschrift, 14, 143-146.

136. ANTON, G. (1914-1915) 'Verschlechterung der Erblichkeit bei Trinkern.' ['Worsening of nausea in drinkers.'] Die Alkoholfrage (Berlin), 11 (New Series, Vol. 5), 242-245.

137. ARCAS, R., JIMENEZ, R., and CRUZ, M. (1978) 'Síndrome alcohólico fetal.' Archives de Pediatrie, 29, 147.

138. ARLITT, A.H. (1919) 'The effect of alcohol upon the intelligent behavior of the white rat and its progeny.' Psychological Monographs, 26, 1-50.

139. ARLITT, A.H., and WELLS, H.G. (1917) 'The effect of alcohol on the reproductive tissues.' Journal of Experimental Medicine, 26, 769-782.

140. ARNAUDOVA, R., and KACVULOV, A. (1978) 'Kafe i bremennost.' ['Coffee and pregnancy.'] Akusherstvo i Ginekologiia (Moscow), 17, 57-61.

141. ARON, E., FLANZY, M., COMBESCOT, C., PUISAIS, J., DEMARET, J.,
      REYNOUARD-BRAULT, F., and IGERT, C. (1965) 'L'alcool est-
      il dans le vin l'élément qui perturbe, chez la ratte, le
      cycle vaginal?' ['Is alcohol the element in wine which dis-
      turbs the estrous cycle in the rat?'] Bulletin de l'Acad-
      émie Nationale de Médicine, 149, 112-120.

142. ARONSSON, M., CARLSSON, C., JOHANSSON, P.R., KYLLERMAN, M.,
      OLEGÅRD, R., SABEL, K.G., and SANDIN, B. (1977) 'Alcohol
      och graviditet.' ['Alcohol during pregnancy.'] Läkartid-
      ningen (Stockholm), 74, 3074-3080.

143. ARRIVE, R. (1899) 'Influence de l'alcoolisme sur la depopu-
      lation.' ['Influence of alcoholism on depopulation.']
      Thèse, Paris.

144. ARULANANTHAM, K., and GOLDSTEIN, G. (1979) 'Neural tube defects
      with fetal alcohol syndrome--reply.' [Letter.] Journal of
      Pediatrics, 95, 329.

145. ASCHKENASY-LELU, P. (1958) 'Action des boissons alcoolisées sur
      le rendement reproducteur du rat.' ['Effect of alcoholic
      beverages on reproduction in the rat.'] Comptes Rendus des
      Seances de l'Académie des Sciences (Paris), 246, 1275-1277.

146. ASCHKENASY-LELU, P. (1958) 'Action d'un oestrogene sur la con-
      sommation spontanée d'une boisson alcoolisée chez le rat.'
      ['The action of estrogen on the spontaneous consumption of
      an alcoholic beverage by the rat.'] Comptes Rendus des
      Seances de l'Académie des Sciences (Paris), 247, 1044-1047.

147. ASHLEY, M.J. (1979) 'Drinking by mothers-to-be: A discussion
      for public health professionals.' Information Review
      (Toronto), pp. 1-7.

148. ASHLEY, M.J. (1981) 'Alcohol use during pregnancy: A challenge
      for the 80's.' Canadian Medical Association Journal, 125,
      141-143.

149. ATHANASIOU, R., SHAVER, P., and TAVRIS, C. (1970) 'Sex: A
      Psychology Today report on more than 20,000 responses to
      101 questions on sexual attitudes and practices.' Psych-
      ology Today, 4, 39.

150. AUROUX, M. (1973) 'Influence, chez le rat, de la nutrition de
      la mère sur le developpment tardif du systeme nerveux cen-
      tral de la progeniture.' ['Influence on the rat of the
      mother's nutrition on the late development of the central
      nervous system of the offspring.'] Comptes Rendus des
      Seances de la Société de Biologie et de ses Filiales (Paris),
      167, 626-629.

151. AUROUX, M., and DEHAUPAS, M.   (1970)   'Influence de la nutrition
         de la mère sur le developpment tardif du systeme nerveux cen-
         tral de la progeniture.'   ['Influence of the mother's nutri-
         tion on the late development of the central nervous system
         in the offspring.']   Comptes Rendus des Seances de la Société
         de Biologie et de ses Filiales (Paris), 164, 1432-1436.

152. AYROMLOOI, J., TOBIAS, M., BERG, P.D., and DESIDERIO, D.   (1979)
         'Effects of ethanol on the circulation and acid-base balance
         of pregnant sheep.'   Obstetrics and Gynecology, 54, 624-630.

B

153. BADEN, J., and SIMMON, V. (1980) 'Mutagenic effects of in-
      halational anesthetics.' Mutation Research, 75, 169-189.

154. BADR, F.M., and BADR, R.S. (1975) 'Induction of dominant lethal
      mutation in male mice by ethyl alcohol.' Nature (London),
      253, 134-136.

155. BADR, F.M., BADR, R.S., and ASKER, R.L., and HUSSAIN, F.H.
      (1977) 'Evaluation of the mutagenic effects of ethyl alco-
      hol by different techniques.' Advances in Experimental Med-
      icine and Biology, 85A, 25-46.

156. BADR, F.M., and BARTKE, A. (1974) 'Effect of ethyl alcohol on
      plasma testosterone level in mice.' Steroids, 23, 921-927.

157. BADR, F.M., BARTKE, A., DALTERIO, S., and BULGER, W. (1977)
      'Suppression of testosterone production by ethyl alcohol:
      Possible mode of action.' Steroids, 30, 647-655.

158. BADR, F.M., SMITH, M.S., DALTERIO, S.L., and BARTKE, A. (1979)
      'Role of the pituitary and the adrenals in mediating the
      effects of alcohol on testicular steroidogenesis in mice.'
      Steroids, 34, 477-482.

159. BAER, D.S., and CRUMPACKER, D.W. (1975) 'Effects of maternal
      ingestion of alcohol on maternal care and behavior on
      progeny in mice.' Behavior Genetics, 5, 88-89.

160. BAER, D.S., and CRUMPACKER, D.W. (1976) 'Fertility and off-
      spring survival in mice selected for different sensitivities
      to alcohol.' Behavior Genetics, 7, 95-103.

161. BALLANTYNE, J.W. (1917) 'Alcohol and antenatal child welfare.'
      British Journal of Inebriety, 14, 93-116.

162. BALLESTA, F., and CRUZ, M. (1978) 'Sindrome alcoholico fetal y
      alteraciones cromosomicas.' ['Fetal alcohol syndrome and
      chromosome alterations.'] Archives de Pediatria, 29, 435-
      443.

163. BANERJEE, U. (1975) 'Conditioned learning in young rats born of
      drug-addicted parents and raised on addictive drugs.'
      Psychopharmacologia (Berlin), 41, 113-116.

164. BARIĆ, L., and MAC ARTHUR, C. (1977) 'Health norms in pregnan-
      cy.' British Journal of Preventive and Social Medicine
      (London), 31, 30-38.

165. BARIĆ, L., MAC ARTHUR, C., and SHERWOOD, M. (1976) 'A study of
      health education aspects of smoking in pregnancy.' Inter-
      national Journal of Health Education (Geneva), 19, 1-16.

166. BARILYAK, I.R., KOZACHUK, S.Y., TSYPKUN, A.G., and ANDRASHKO, V.V.
      (1980) 'Functional state of the central nervous system in
      rats subjected to the effect of ethanol in the antenatal
      period.' Doklady Akademii Nauk Ukraine USSR, Ser. B,
      Geologiya, Khimiya I Biologiya Nauki 0, 69-72.

167. BARK, N. (1979) 'Fertility and offspring of alcoholic women:
      An unsuccessful search for the fetal alcohol syndrome.'
      British Journal of Addiction (Edinburgh), 74, 43-49.

168. BARNES, D.E., and WALKER, D.W. (1980) 'Neuronal loss in hippo-
      campus and cerebellar cortex in rats prenatally exposed to
      ethanol.' Alcoholism: Clinical and Experimental Research,
      4, 209 (abstract).

169. BARNES, D.E., and WALKER, D.W. (1981) 'Prenatal ethanol exposure
      permanently reduces the number of pyrimidal neurons in rat
      hippocampus.' Developmental Brain Research, 1, 3-24.

170. BARNES, F.H. (1915) 'Heredity in alcoholism.' Long Island
      Medical Journal, 9, 337-341.

171. BARR, H.M., STREISSGUTH, A.P., and MARTIN, D.C. (1980) 'Re-
      lationship of social drinking during pregnancy to growth of
      infants at 8 months.' Alcoholism: Clinical and Experimen-
      tal Research, 4, 210 (abstract).

172. BARRADA, M.I., VIRNIG, N.L., EDWARDS, L.E., and HAKANSON, E.Y.
      (1977) 'Maternal intravenous ethanol in the prevention of
      respiratory distress syndrome.' American Journal of Obstet-
      rics and Gynecology, 129, 25-30.

173. BARRY, R.G.G., and O'NUALLAIN, S. (1975) 'Case report: Foetal
      alcoholism. St. Finbarr's Hospital.' Irish Journal of Med-
      ical Science (Dublin), 144, 286-288.

174. BARTLE, W.R., and PATON, T.W. (1978) 'Effects of drugs during
      pregnancy.' Modern Medicine of Canada, 33, 30-38.

175. BARTLETT, D., and DAVIS, A. (1980) 'Recognizing fetal alcohol
      syndrome in the nursery.' JOGN Nursing, 9, 223-225.

176. BARTOLI, G. (1980) 'Children as victims of alcohol.' Revue
      de l'Infirmiere, 30, 48-49.

177 BARTOSHESKY, L.E., FEINGOLD, M., SCHEINER, A.P., and DONOVAN, C.M.
         (1979) 'A paternal fetal alcohol syndrome and fetal alcohol
         syndrome in a child whose alcoholic parents had stopped
         drinking.' Proceedings of the Birth Defects Conference
         (sponsored by Northwestern University/National Foundation
         March of Dimes), Chicago, Illinois (June 24-27).

178. BAUER-MOFFETT, C., and ALTMAN, J. (1975) 'Ethanol-induced
         reductions in cerebellar growth of infant rats.' Experi-
         mental Neurology, 48, 378-382.

179. BAUER-MOFFETT, C., and ALTMAN, J. (1977) 'The effect of ethanol
         chronically administered to preweanling rats on cerebellar
         development: A morphological study.' Brain Research,
         (Amsterdam), 119, 249-268.

180. BEATTIE, J.O. (1981) 'Alcohol and the fetal brain.' [Letter.]
         Lancet (London), 1, 788.

181. BEAUMONT, T. (1842) 'Remarks made in opposition to the views
         of Dr. Clutterbuck.' Lancet (London), 2, 340-343.

182. BECK, K.J., and HINCKERS, H.J. (1972) 'Untersuchungen über den
         Übertritt von Alkohol in den Zervikalmukus und seine Be-
         deutung für die Sterilität der Frau.' ['Study on the passage
         of alcohol into the cervical mucus and its role in sterility
         of the woman.'] Geburtshilfe und Frauenheilkunde (Stutt-
         gart), 32, 585-589.

183. BECKER, B.A. (1975) 'Teratogens.' In: Toxicology, The Basic
         Science of Poisons. New York: Macmillan Publishing Company,
         pp. 313-331.

184. BECKMAN, L.J. (1978) 'Sex-role conflict in alcoholic women:
         Myth or reality.' Journal of Abnormal Psychology, 87, 408-
         417.

185. BECKMAN, L.J. (1979) 'Reported effects of alcohol on the sex-
         ual feelings and behavior of women alcoholics and nonalco-
         holics.' Journal of Studies on Alcohol, 40, 272-282.

186. BEECHER, L. (1827) Six Sermons on the Nature, Occasions, Signs,
         Evils, and Remedy of Intemperance. Boston: Crocker and
         Brewster.

187. BEEK, B., and OBE, G. (1975) 'The human leukocyte test system.
         VI. The use of sister chromatid exchange as possible indi-
         cators for mutagenic activities.' Humangenetik (Berlin),
         29, 127-134.

188. BELFER, M.L., SHADER, R.I., CARROLL, M., and HARMATZ, J.S. (1971)
         'Alcoholism in women.' Archives of General Psychiatry, 25,
         540-544.

189. BELILES, R.P. (1972) 'The influence of pregnancy on the acute
      toxicity of various compounds in mice.' Toxicology and Ap-
      plied Pharmacology, 23, 537-540.

190. BELINKOFF, S., and HALL, O.W., JR. (1950) 'Intravenous alcohol
      during labor.' American Journal of Obstetrics and Gyne-
      cology, 59, 429-432.

191. BENEDIK, T.G. (1972) 'Food and drink as aphrodisiacs.' Sexual
      Behavior, 2, 5-10.

192. BERENSON, D. (1976) 'Sexual counseling with alcoholics.' In:
      Sexual Counseling for Persons with Alcohol Problems: Pro-
      ceedings of a Workshop. Ed. J. Newman. Western Pennsyl-
      vania Institute of Alcohol Studies, University of Pitts-
      burgh.

193. BERGSTROM, R.M., SAINIO, K., and TAALAS, J. (1967) 'The effect
      of ethanol on the EEG of the guinea pig foetus.' Medicina
      et Pharmacologia Experimentalis, 16, 448-452.

194. BERKOWITZ, G.S. (1981) 'An epidemiologic study of preterm
      delivery.' American Journal of Epidemiology, 113, 81-92.

195. BERKOWITZ, G., HOLFORD, T., KASL, S., and KELSEY, J. (1979)
      'The epidemiology of pre-term delivery.' American Journal
      of Epidemiology, 110, 355 (abstract).

196. BERTHOLET, E. (1909) 'De l'influence de l'alcoolisme chronique
      sur le testicule humaine.' ['The influence of chronic alco-
      holism on the human testicle.'] The Proceedings of the
      Twelfth International Conference on Alcoholism (London), 12,
      294-298.

197. BERTHOLET, E. (1909) 'Über Atrophie des Hodens bei chronischem
      Alkoholismus.' ['Regarding the atrophy of the testicle in
      chronic alcoholism.'] Zentralblatt für Allgemeine Path-
      ologie und Pathologische Anatomie (Jena), 20, 1062-1066.

198. BERTHOLET, E. (1912) 'Alterations anatomo-pathologique, obser-
      vées à l'autopsie de 100 alcoolique chroniques.' ['Anatomo-
      pathological alterations, observed in the autopsy of 100
      chronic alcoholics.'] In: Bericht über den XIII. Inter-
      nationalen Kongress gegen den Alkoholismus (The Hague), 13,
      181-186.

199. BERTHOLET, F. (1913) Action de l'alcoolisme chronique sur les
      organes de l'homme et sur les glandes reporcutives en par-
      ticular. [The action of chronic alcoholism on the organs of
      the male and on the reproductive glands in particular.]
      Lausanne.

200. BERTHOLET, F. (1914) Heredité et alcoolisme. [Heredity and
      Alcoholism.] Lausanne.

201. BESKID, M. (1979) 'Histochemical and morphological evaluation of cerebral cortex of newborn rat in the course of joint ethanol and pyrazole administration.' Acta Histochemica, 64, 89-97.

202. BESKID, M., KOWALIK, J., and MACIEJCZYK, W. (1978) 'Ethanol toxic effect on the newborn rat liver: Histochemical and electron-microscopal investigations.' Experimentelle Pathologie (Jena), 15, 355-360.

203. BESKID, M., MAJDECKI, T., and SKLADZINSKI, J. (1975) 'The effect of ethanol applied during gestation on the mitochondria of the hepatic cells of pups.' Folia Histochemica et Cytochemica (Krakow), 13, 175-180.

204. BESKID, M., and TLALKA, J. (1980) 'Wpływ etanolu na płod.' ['Effect of alcohol on the fetus.'] Problemy Alkoholizmu (Warsaw), 27, 9-10.

205. BESSEY, W.E. (1872) 'On the use of alcoholic stimulants by nursing mothers.' Canadian Medical Record, 1, 195-200.

206. BESSIÈRE, E., and BERGOUIGNAN, M. (1945) 'Ptosis congenital familial, suivi d'aggravation tardive chez une hérédo-alcoolique.' Journale de Médicine Bordeaux, 121-122, 497-498.

207. BEVERAGE ALCOHOL INFORMATION COUNCIL. (1979) 'Public education program on drinking and pregnancy.' Washington, D.C.

208. BEYERS, N., and MOOSA, A. (1978) 'The fetal alcohol syndrome, case reports.' South Africa Medical Journal (Cape Town), 54, 575-578.

209. BEZZOLA, D. (1901) 'A statistical investigation into the role of alcohol in the origin of innate imbecility.' Quarterly Journal of Inebriety, 23, 346-354.

210. BEZZOLA, D. (1902) 'Statistische Untersuchungen über die Rolle des Alkohols bei der Entstehung des originaren Schwachsinns.' ['Statistical studies regarding the role of alcohol in the condition of original pregnancy.'] In: Bericht über den VIII. Internationalen Kongress gegen den Alkoholismus (Vienna), pp. 109-111.

211. BHALLA, V.K., CHEN, C.J.H., and GNANAPRAKASAM, M.S. (1979) 'Effects of in vivo administration of human chorionic gonadotropin and ethanol on the processes of testicular receptor depletion and replenishment.' Life Sciences (Oxford), 24, 1315-1323.

212. BIANCHINE, J.W., and TAYLOR, B.D. (1974) 'Response to "Noonan syndrome and fetal alcohol syndrome" by B.D. Hall and W.A. Orenstein.' Lancet (London), 1, 933.

213. BIENIARZ, J., BURD, L., MOTEW, M., and SCOMMEGNA, A.   (1971)
      'Inhibition of uterine contractivity in labor.' American
      Journal of Obstetrics and Gynecology, 3, 874-885.

214. BIERICH, J.R.   (1978) 'Pränatale Schädigungen durch Alkohol.'
      ['Prenatal damages from alcohol.'] Der Internist (Berlin),
      19, 131-139.

215. BIERICH, J.R.   (1980) 'Fetal alcohol syndrome.' Deutsche Med-
      izinische Wochenschrift, 105, 1340.

216. BIERICH, J.R., and MAJEWSKI, F.   (1977) 'Alkoholbedingte Embryo-
      pathie.' ['Alcohol-induced embryopathy.'] Jahrestagung
      1977 der Deutschen Gesellschaft für Verkehrsmedizin (Ham-
      burg), pp. 20-22.

217. BIERICH, J.R., MAJEWSKI, F., MICHAELIS, R., and TILLNER, I.
      (1976) 'Über das embryo-fetale Alkoholsyndrom.' ['On the
      embryofetal alcohol syndrome.'] European Journal of Ped-
      iatrics, 121, 155-177.

218. BILSKI, F.   (1921) 'Über Blastophorie durch Alkohol.' ['Re-
      garding blastophoria through alcohol.'] Archiv für Ent-
      wicklungmechanik der Organismen (Leipzig), 47, 627-651.

219. BINKIEWICZ, A., ROBINSON, M.J., and SENIOR, B.   (1978) 'Pseudo-
      Cushing syndrome caused by alcohol in breast milk.' Jour-
      nal of Pediatrics, 93, 965-967.

220. BISDOM, C.J.W.   (1936) 'Alkohol- en nicotinevergiftiging bij
      zuigelingen.' ['Alcohol and nicotine poisoning in off-
      spring.'] Mündschrift Kindergenese, 6, 332-341.

221. BISSONNETTE, J.M., CRONAN, J.Z., RICHARDS, L.L., and WICKHAM, W.K.
      (1979) 'Placental transfer of water and nonelectrolytes
      during a single circulatory passage.' American Journal of
      Physiology, 236, C47-C52.

222. BLAKE, C.A.   (1974) 'Centrally acting drugs must inhibit spon-
      taneous neural stimulation of luteinizing hormone release
      for a specific 7-hour period to block ovulation in rats.'
      Federation Proceedings; Federation of American Societies for
      Experimental Biology, 33 (Part I), 221 (abstract).

223. BLAKE, C.A.   (1974) 'Differentiation between the "critical per-
      iod," the "activation period" and the "potential activation
      period" for neurohumoral stimulation of LH release in pro-
      estrous rats.' Endocrinology, 95, 572-578.

224. BLAKE, C.A.   (1974) 'Localization of the inhibitory actions of
      ovulation-blocking drugs on release of luteinizing hormone
      in ovariectomized rats.' Endocrinology, 95, 999-1004.

225. BLAKE, C.A.   (1978)   'Paradoxical effects of drugs acting on the central nervous system on the preovulatory release of pituitary luteinizing hormone in pro-oestrous rats.' Journal of Endocrinology, 79, 319-326.

226. BLEICHER, S.J., and WALTMAN, R.   (1970)   'Ethanol infusions.' Lancet (London), 1, 1404.

227. BLIGNAUT, F.W.   (1958)   Enkele Aspekte van die Alkoholvebruik Deur die Witmuis in die Laboratorium. [Individual Aspects of Alcohol Use in Laboratory Mice.] Pretoria: Communications of the University of South Africa.

228. BLIGNAUT, F.W.   (1965)   'Alcohol and functional processes.' Communications of the University of South Africa, Series C, 55, 1-18.

229. BLINICK, G., WALLACH, R.C., JEREZ, E., and ACKERMAN, B.D.   (1976) 'Drug addiction in pregnancy and the neonate.' American Journal of Obstetrics and Gynecology, 125, 135-142.

230. BLUHM, A.   (1930)   'Zum Problem "Alkohol und Nachkommenschaft."' ['Regarding the Problem "Alcohol and Pregnancy."'] Archiv für Rassen und Gesamte Biologie, 24, 12-18.

231. BLUHM, A.   (1930)   Zum Problem "Alkohol und Nachkommenschaft." [Regarding the Problem "Alcohol and Pregnancy."] Munich: J.F. Lehmann.

232. BLUME, S.B.   (1980)   'Translating research into public policy: Prevention of fetal alcohol syndrome in New York State.' Teratology, 21, 28A (abstract). [Also in Neurobehavioral Toxicology, 2, 285-286.]

233. BLUME, S.B.   (1981)   'Drinking and pregnancy: Preventing fetal alcohol syndrome.' New York State Journal of Medicine, 81, 95-98.

234. BO, W.J., KRUEGER, W.A., RUDEEN, P.K., and SYMMES, S.K.   (1981 'The effect of different doses of ethanol on ovarian function.' Alcoholism: Clinical and Experimental Research, 5, 349 (abstract).

235. BOCK, J.   (1979)   'Closeup on fetal alcohol syndrome.' Canadian Nurse, 75, 35.

236. BOGGAN, W.O.   (1980)   'Effects of alcohol and barbiturates in combination.' Paper presented at the Fetal Alcohol Syndrome Workshop, Seattle, Washington (May 2-4).

237. BOGGAN, W.O.   (1981)   'Animal models of the fetal alcohol syndrome.' In: Fetal Alcohol Syndrome. Volume 3: Animal Studies. Ed. E.L. Abel. Boca Raton, Florida: CRC Press (in press).

238. BOGGAN, W.O. (1981) 'Effect of prenatal ethanol exposure on
     neurochemical systems.' In: Fetal Alcohol Syndrome.
     Volume 3: Animal Studies. Ed. E.L. Abel. Boca Raton,
     Florida: CRC Press (in press).

239. BOGGAN, W.O., and RANDALL, C.L. (1980) 'Effect of low-dose pre-
     natal alcohol exposure on behavior and the response to alco-
     hol.' Alcoholism: Clinical and Experimental Research, 4,
     226 (abstract).

240. BOGGAN, W.O., and RANDALL, C.L. (1980) 'Studies on the effects
     of prenatal ethanol exposure in C57BL mice.' Teratology,
     21, 28A-29A (abstract).

241. BOGGAN, W.O., RANDALL, C.L., and DEBEUKELAER, M. (1978) 'Renal
     abnormalities in mice prenatally exposed to ethanol.' Paper
     presented at National Alcoholism Forum, St. Louis, Missouri.

242. BOGGAN, W.O., RANDALL, C.L., DEBEUKELAER, M., and SMITH, R.
     (1978) 'Renal anomalies in mice prenatally exposed to eth-
     anol.' Alcoholism: Clinical and Experimental Research, 2,
     201 (abstract).

243. BOGGAN, W.O., RANDALL, C.L, DEBEUKELAER, M., and SMITH, R.
     (1979) 'Renal anomalies in mice prenatally exposed to eth-
     anol.' Research Communications in Chemical Pathology and
     Pharmacology, 23, 127-142.

244. BOGGAN, W.O., RANDALL, C.L., and DODDS, H.M. (1979) 'Delayed
     sexual maturation in female $C_{57}BL/6J$ mice prenatally exposed
     to alcohol.' Research Communications in Chemical Pathology
     and Pharmacology, 23, 117-125.

245. BOGGAN, W.O., RANDALL, C.L., WILSON-BURROWS, C., and PARKER, L.S.
     (1979) 'Effect of prenatal ethanol on brain serotonergic
     systems.' Transactions of the American Society of Neuro-
     chemistry, 10, 186.

246. BOND, N.W. (1978) 'Fetal alcohol syndrome.' Medical Journal of
     Australia (Sydney), 65, 164.

247. BOND, N.W. (1979) 'Effects of postnatal alcohol exposure on
     maternal nesting behavior on the rat.' Physiological Psy-
     chology, 4, 396-398.

248. BOND, N.W. (1980) 'Postnatal alcohol exposure in the rat: Hebb-
     Williams maze performance, maternal behavior, and pup devel-
     opment.' Physiological Psychology, 8, 437-443.

249. BOND, N.W. (1981) 'Effects of prenatal ethanol exposure on
     avoidance conditioning in high- and low-avoidance rat
     strains.' Psychopharmacology (Berlin), 74, 177-181.

250. BOND, N.W., and DIGIUSTO, E.L. (1976) 'Effects of prenatal al-
     cohol consumption on open-field behavior and alcohol prefer-
     ence in rats.' Psychopharmacology (Berlin), 46, 163-168.

251. BOND, N.W., and DIGIUSTO, E.L. (1977) 'Effects of prenatal alcohol consumption on shock avoidance learning in rats.' Psychological Reports, 41, 1269-1270.

252. BOND, N.W., and DIGIUSTO, E.L. (1977) 'Prenatal alcohol consumption and open-field behaviour in rats: Effects of age at time of testing.' Psychopharmacology (Berlin), 52, 311-312.

253. BOND, N.W., and DIGIUSTO, E.L. (1978) 'Avoidance conditioning and Hebb-Williams maze performance in rats treated prenatally with alcohol.' Psychopharmacology (Berlin), 58, 69-71.

254. BONHOFFER, K. (1906) 'Chronischer Alkoholismus und Vererbung.' ['Chronic alcoholism and heredity.'] Alkoholismus, New Series, 3, 297-305.

255. BONN, B.G. (1978) 'Alcohol and the fetus.' Maryland State Medical Journal, 27, 21-23.

256. BONNIE, R.J. (1980) 'Regulation of alcohol, tobacco, and other drugs: The agenda for law reform.' National Institute of Drug Abuse Research Monograph Series, 34, 272-286.

257. BONTA, M., and CZEIZEL, E. (1980) 'A terhesség és szülés alatti alkohol-therapie, mint iatrogénártalom forrása.' ['Alcohol therapy during pregnancy and labor as a source of iatrogenic damage.'] [Letter.] Orvosi Hetilap, 121, 1665.

258. BORGMAN, R.F., and WARDLAW, F.B. (1977) 'Influence of maternal ethanol consumption in rats upon the dams and the offspring.' South Carolina Agricultural Experimental Station Technical Bulletin, 597, 1-17.

259. BORGSTEDT, A.D., and ROSEN, M.G. (1968) 'Medication during labor correlated with behavior and EEG of the newborn.' American Journal of Diseases of Children, 115, 21-24.

260. BORKOWSKA, U. (1979) 'Liczba PUW wśród dzieci powiatu pułtuskiego.' ['Decayed, missing, or filled teeth index in children in the County of Pułtusk.'] Czasopismo Stomatologiczne, 32, 449-452.

261. BORLÉE, I., and LECHAT, M.F. (1978) 'Résultats d'une enquête sur les malformations congénitales dans le Hainaut.' ['Results of a survey on congenital malformations in Hainaut.'] Archives Belges de Médicine Sociale, Hygiene, Médicine du Travail et Médicine Legale, 36, 77-99.

262. BORLÉE, I., LECHAT, M.F., BOUCKAERT, A., and COLTRO, A. (1977) 'Regional survey on congenital malformations: Methodology and organization.' Louvain Médical, 96, 121-134.

263. BORTERYU, J.P.   (1967)   'La toxicomanie alcoolique parentale et
     les repercussions sur la descendance.'   ['Prenatal alcohol
     addiction and its effects on offspring.']   Ph.D. Thesis,
     University of Nantes, France.

264. BOSTON CITY HOSPITAL.   (1914)   Fiftieth Annual Report of Trus-
     tees.   February 1, 1913, to January 31, 1914, pp. 40 et
     passim.

265. BOSTRÖM, H.   (1979)   'Foetopathy caused by alcohol: A critical
     review.'   In: Metabolic Effects of Alcohol: Proceedings of
     the International Symposium on Metabolic Effects of Alcohol
     (Milan, June 18-21).   Ed. P. Avogaro, C.R. Sirtori, and
     E. Tremoli.   New York: Elsevier, pp. 49-54.

266. BOUIN, P., and GARNIER, C.   (1900)   'Alterations du tube sémini-
     fère au cours de l'alcoolisme experimental chez le rat
     blanc.'   ['Alterations in the seminiferous tubule in the
     course of experimental alcoholism in the white rat.']
     Comptes Rendus des Seances de la Société de Biologie
     et de ses Filiales (Paris), 52, 23.

267. BOYDEN, T.W., SILVERT, M.A., and PAMENTER, R.W.   (1981)   'Acetal-
     dehyde acutely impairs canine testicular testosterone secre-
     tion.'   European Journal of Pharmacology, 70, 571-576.

268. BRANCHEY, L., and FRIEDHOFF, A.J.   (1973)   'The influence of
     ethanol administered to pregnant rats on tyrosine hydroxylase
     activity of their offspring.'   Psychopharmacologia (Berlin),
     32, 151-156.

269. BRANCHEY, L., and FRIEDHOFF, A.J.   (1976)   'Biochemical and be-
     havioral changes in rats exposed to ethanol in utero.'
     Annals of the New York Academy of Sciences, 273, 328-330.

270. BRANDT, N.J., and MØLLER, J.   (1978)   'Føtalt alkoholsyndrom.'
     ['Fetal alcohol syndrome.']   Ugeskrift for Laeger (Copen-
     hagen), 140, 282-288.

271. BRAUN, R., and SCHÖNEICH, J.   (1975)   'The influence of ethanol
     and carbon tetrachloride on the mutagenic effectivity of
     cyclophosphamide in the host-mediated assay with Salmonella
     typhimurium.'   Mutation Research (Amsterdam), 31, 191-194.

272. BREGMAN, A.A.   (1977)   'Cytogenetic effects of ethanol in human
     leukocyte cultures.'   Environmental Mutagen Society Newslet-
     ter, 4, 35-36.

273. BRENT, R.L.   (1978)   'Vulnerability of the preimplantation mam-
     malian embryo.'   Teratology, 17, 17A (abstract).

274. BRESKIN, M.W., CLARREN, S.K., and LITTLE, R.E.   (1981)   'Zinc
     concentrations in serum and hair and dietary zinc content of
     alcoholic women of child-bearing age compared with suitable
     controls.'   Alcoholism: Clinical and Experimental Research,
     5, 144 (abstract).

275. BRIDDELL, D.W., RIMM, D.C., CADDY, G.R., KRAWITZ, G., SHOLIS, D., and WUNDERLIN, R.J. (1978) 'Effects of alcohol and cognitive set on sexual arousal to deviant stimuli.' Journal of Abnormal Psychology, 87, 418-430.

276. BRIDDELL, D.W., and WILSON, G.T. (1976) 'Effects of alcohol and expectancy set on male sexual arousal.' Journal of Abnormal Psychology, 85, 225-234.

277. BROCK, R.C. (1923) 'Alcohol in relation to race.' Guy's Hospital Gazette (London), 38, 502.

278. BROWN, N.A. (1980) 'Ethanol effects on embryogenesis.' Paper presented at the Fetal Alcohol Syndrome Workshop, Seattle, Washington (May 2-4).

279. BROWN, N.A., GOULDING, E.H., and FABRO, S. (1979) 'Ethanol embryotoxicity: Direct effects on mammalian embryos in vitro.' Science, 206, 573-575.

280. BROZIN-BOHMAN, V., and JOHANSSON, L. (1979) 'Kvinnomissbruk--fosterskador.' ['Women addicts--damage to the fetus.'] Alkohol och Narkotika, 73, 1.

281. BRUNO, F., and FERRACUTI, F. (1977) 'Droga e condotte sessuali.' ['Drugs and sexual behavior.'] Quaderni di Criminolologia Clinica (Rome), 19, 17-36.

282. BRZEK, A. (1977) 'Male sexuality and alcohol.' Casopis Lekaru Ceskych 116, 1024-1026.

283. BRZEK, A., SKALÁ, J. and LACHMAN, M. (1978) 'Spermabefunde bei Alkoholikern.' ['Spermatologic findings in alcoholics.'] Dermatologische Monatsschrift (Leipzig), 164, 557-559.

284. BRZEK, A., SKALÁ, J., and LACHMAN, M. (1980) 'Změny spermatologických nálezů během protialkoholní léčby.' ['Spermatologic parameter changes in the course of alcoholism treatment.'] Protialkoholicky Obzor (Bratislava), 15, 15-18.

285. BRZECKA, K., WACHNIK, S., and WIERCINSKI, J. (1977) 'Narażenie płodu na etanol w oparciu o jego rozprzestrzenianie się u kobiet ciężarnych.' ['Exposure of the fetus to ethanol estimated on the basis of the rate of alcohol distribution in a pregnant woman.'] Problemy Alkoholizmu (Warsaw), 24, 5-6.

286. BUCHET, J.P., ROELS, H., HUBERMONT, G., and LAUWERYS, R. (1978) 'Placental transfer of lead, mercury, cadmium, and carbon monoxide in women. 2. Influence of some epidemiological factors on the frequency distributions of the biological indices in maternal and umbilical cord blood.' Environmental Research, 15, 494-503.

287. BUCKALEW, L.W. (1977) 'Developmental and behavioral effects of
      maternal and fetal/neonatal alcohol exposure.' Research
      Communications in Psychology, Psychiatry, and Behavior, 2,
      179-191.

288. BUCKALEW, L.W. (1978) 'Effect of maternal alcohol consumption
      during nursing on offspring activity.' Research Communica-
      tions in Psychology, Psychiatry, and Behavior, 3, 353-358.

289. BUCKALEW, L.W. (1978) 'Problems in use of rodents for studies of
      maternal exposure to alcohol.' Psychological Reports, 43,
      1313-1314.

290. BUCKALEW, L.W. (1979) 'Alcohol preference, housing effect and
      bottle position effect in maternally-exposed offspring.'
      Addictive Behaviors (Oxford), 4, 275-277.

291. BUEHLER, B. (1978) 'Fetal alcohol syndrome.' UNA Communique,
      5, 11.

292. BUFFINGTON, V., MARTIN, D.C., and STREISSGUTH, A.P. (1980) 'Slow
      cortical potentials in the fetal alcohol syndrome.' Psycho-
      physiology (in press).

293. BUFFINGTON, V., MARTIN, D.C., STREISSGUTH, A.P., and SMITH, D.W.
      (1981) 'Contingent negative variation in the fetal alcohol
      syndrome: A preliminary report.' Neurobehavioral Toxicol-
      ogy and Teratology, 3, 183-185.

294. BURKE, J.P., and FENTON, M.R. (1978) 'The effect of maternal
      ethanol consumption on aldehyde dehydrogenase activity in
      neonates.' Research Communications in Psychology, Psy-
      chiatry, and Behavior, 3, 169-172.

295. BURNS, R.E., NIPPO, M.M., and GRAY, H.G. (1980) 'The fetal al-
      cohol syndrome in rats.' Journal of Animal Science, 51,
      188-189.

296. BURROWS, G.N., and FERRIS, T.F. (1975) Medical Complications
      during Pregnancy. Philadelphia: Saunders.

297. BURSEY, R.G. (1973) 'Effect of maternal ethanol consumption
      during gestation and lactation on the development and
      learning performance of the offspring.' Ph.D. Thesis,
      Clemson University, Clemson, South Carolina.

298. BURTON, G., and KAPLAN, H.M. (1968) 'Sexual behavior and ad-
      justment of married alcoholics.' Quarterly Journal of
      Studies on Alcoholism, 29, 603-609.

299. BURTON, R. (1906; Orig. 1621) The Anatomy of Melancholy.
      Volume 1, Part I, Section 2: 'Causes of melancholy.'
      London: William Tegg.

300. BUSH, P.J. (1980) Drugs, Alcohol, and Sex. New York: Rich-
      ard Marek Publishers.

301. BUTLER, M.G., SANGER, W.G., and VEOMETT, G.E. (1981) 'Increased
      frequency of sister-chromatid exchanges in alcoholics.'
      Mutation Research (Amsterdam), 85, 71-76.

302. BUTTAR, H.S. (1980) 'Effects of the combined administration of
      ethanol and chlordiazepoxide on the pre- and postnatal
      development of rats.' Neurobehavioral Toxicology, 2, 217-
      225. [Also in Teratology, 21, 32A-33A (abstract).]

303. BYRNE, J.M. (1980) 'Animal models of the fetal alcohol syn-
      drome.' In: An Assessment of Statistics on Alcohol-Related
      Problems. Prepared for the Distilled Spirits Council of the
      United States. (Paged by sections.) [Washington, D.C.],
      pages II-1-II-14.

C

304. CADOTTE, M., ALLARD, S., and VERDY, M. (1973) 'Lack of effect of ethanol in vitro on human chromosomes.' Annales de Genetique (Paris), 16: 55-56.

305. CAHUANA, A., KRAUEL, J., MOLINA, V., LIZÁRRAGA, I., and ALFONSO, H. (1977) 'Fetopatía alcohólica.' ['Alcohol fetopathy.'] Anales Espanoles de Pediatria (Madrid), 10, 673-676.

306. CAMPBELL, M.A., and FANTEL, A.G. (1981) 'Effect of ethanol consumption on the teratogenic bioactivation of cyclophosphamide in vitro.' Teratology, 23, 30A (abstract).

307. CARDEN, J.H. (1977) 'Alcool, grosse et morbidité feto-infantile.' ['Alcohol, pregnancy, and fetal-infantile morbidity.'] Revue de l'Alcoolisme (Paris), 23, 201-210.

308. CARITIS, S.N., EDELSTONE, D.I., and MUELLER-HEUBACH, E. (1979) 'Pharmacologic inhibition of preterm labor.' American Journal of Obstetrics and Gynecology, 133, 557-578.

309. CARPENTER, J.A., and ARMENTI, N.P. (1972) 'Some effects of ethanol on human sexual and aggressive behavior.' In: The Biology of Alcoholism. Volume 2: Physiology and Behavior. Ed. B. Kissin and H. Begleiter. New York: Plenum Press, pp. 509-543.

310. CARVER, J.W., NASH, J.B., EMERSON, G.A., and MOORE, W.T. (1953) 'Effects of pregnancy and lactation on voluntary alcohol intake of hamsters.' Federation Proceedings; Federation of American Societies for Experimental Biology, 12, 309.

311. CASTRÉN, O., GUMMERUS, M., and SAARIKOSKI, S. (1975) 'Treatment of imminent premature labour: A comparison between the effects of nylidrin chloride and isoxuprine chloride as well as of ethanol.' Acta Obstetrica et Gynecologica Scandinavica (Lund), 54, 95-100.

312. CATZ, C.S., and ABUELO, D. (1974) 'Drugs and pregnancy.' Drug Therapy, 4, 79-80.

313. CAUL, W.F., FERNANDEZ, K., and MICHAELIS, R.C. (1980) 'Discrim-
        ination acquisition and reversal following prenatal ethanol
        exposure.' Paper presented at the International Society for
        Developmental Psychobiology, Cincinnati, Ohio (November 8).

314. CAUL, W.F., OSBORNE, G.L., FERNANDEZ, K., and HENDERSON, G.I.
        (1978) 'Prenatal ethanol effects on development and adult
        open-field and avoidance performance in rats.' Alcoholism:
        Clinical and Experimental Research, 2, 216.

315. CAUL, W.F., OSBORNE, G.L., FERNANDEZ, K., and HENDERSON, G.I.
        (1979) 'Open-field and avoidance performance of rats as a
        function of prenatal ethanol treatment.' Addictive Behav-
        iors (Oxford), 4, 311-322.

316. CAUSSADE, L., NEIMANN, N., and BLANE, H. (1940) 'Fails relatifs
        à l'alcoolisme infantile.' ['Failures relating to infantile
        alcoholism.'] Pédiatrie (Lyons), 38, 531-535.

317. CAVENER, D.R., and CLEGG, M.T. (1978) 'Dynamics of correlated
        genetic systems. IV. Multilocus effects of ethanol stress
        environments.' Genetics, 90, 629-644.

318. CAYROCHE, P., MARIANI, P., CARNOT, J.F., SAIGNES, F., and GUIL-
        LON, C. (1979) 'Syndromes et maladies rares ou peu con-
        nus. L'embryofoetopathie alcoolique. À propos de cinq
        nouvelles observations.' ['Rare or little-known syndromes
        and illnesses: The fetal alcohol syndrome; 5 new obser-
        vations.'] Médecine Infantile, 86, 541-555.

319. CENI, C. (1904) 'Influenza dell'alcoolismo sul potere di'pro-
        creare e sui discendenti.' ['The influence of alcohol on
        the ability to reproduce and on the descendants.'] Rivista
        Sperimentelle di Freniatria, 30, 339-353.

320. CENTER FOR DISEASE CONTROL, U.S. DEPARTMENT OF HEALTH, EDUCATION,
        AND WELFARE. (1977) 'Fetal alcohol syndrome.' Morbidity
        and Mortality Weekly Report, 26, 178.

321. CHAFETZ, M.E. (1965) Liquor: The Servant of Man. Boston and
        Toronto: Little, Brown, and Co.

322. CHAFETZ, M.E., BLANE, H.T., and HILL, M.J. (1971) 'Children of
        alcoholics: Observations in a child guidance clinic.'
        Quarterly Journal of Studies on Alcohol, 32, 687-698.

323. CHAN, A.W.K., and ABEL, E.L. (1982) 'Absence of long-lasting
        effects of brain receptors for neurotransmitters in rats pre-
        nattaly exposed to alcohol.' Research Communications in Sub-
        stance Abuse, in press.

324. CHAPIN, R.E., BREESE, G.R., and MUELLER, R.A. (1980) 'Possible
        mechanisms of reduction of plasma luteinizing hormone by
        ethanol.' Journal of Pharmacology and Experimental Thera-
        peutics, 212, 6-10.

325.   CHAPMAN, E.R., and WILLIAMS, P.T., JR.   (1951)   'Intravenous
       alcohol as an obstetrical analgesia.'   American Journal of
       Obstetrics and Gynecology, 61, 676-679.

326.   CHAR, F.   (1976)   'Fetal alcohol syndrome with Noonan phenotype.'
       Birth Defects, 12, 81-84.

327.   CHAUDHURY, R.R., and MATTHEWS, M.   (1966)   'Effect of alcohol on
       the fertility of female rabbits.'   Journal of Endocrinology
       (London), 34, 275-276.

328.   CHAUHAN, P.S., ARAVINDAKSHAN, M., KUMAR, N.S., and SUNDARAM, K.
       (1980)   'Failure of ethanol to induce dominant lethal muta-
       tions in Wistar male rats.'   Mutation Research (Amsterdam),
       79, 263-275.

329.   CHEN, J.J., and SMITH, E.R.   (1979)   'Effects of perinatal alco-
       hol on sexual differentiation and open-field behavior in
       rats.'   Hormones and Behavior, 13, 219-231.

330.   CHEN, J.S., RILEY, E.P., and DRISCOLL, C.D.   (1981)   'Ontogeny of
       suckling in rat pups prenatally exposed to ethanol.'   Alco-
       holism: Clinical and Experimental Research, 5, 145 (ab-
       stract).

331.   CHERNOFF, G.F.   (1975)   'A mouse model of the fetal alcohol syn-
       drome.'   Teratology, 11, 14A.

332.   CHERNOFF, G.F.   (1977)   'The fetal alcohol syndrome in mice: An
       animal model.'   Paper presented at the Fetal Alcohol Syn-
       drome Workshop, San Diego, California.

333.   CHERNOFF, G.F.   (1977)   'The fetal alcohol syndrome in mice: An
       animal model.'   Teratology, 15, 223-229.

334.   CHERNOFF, G.F.   (1980)   'Introduction: A teratologist's view of
       the fetal alcohol syndrome.'   In: Currents in Alcoholism.
       Volume 7:   Recent Advances in Research and Treatment.
       Ed. M. Galanter.   New York: Grune and Stratton, pp. 7-13.

335.   CHERNOFF, G.F.   (1980)   'The fetal alcohol syndrome in mice:
       Maternal variables.'   Teratology, 22, 71-75.

336.   CHERNOFF, G.F.   (1981)   'Alcohol teratogenicity: Teratogen-
       genotype interactions.'   Teratology, 23, 31A (abstract).

337.   CHESLER, A., LA BELLE, G.C., and HIMWICH, H.E.   (1942)   'The
       relative effects of toxic doses of alcohol on fetal, newborn
       and adult rats.'   Quarterly Journal of Studies on Alcohol,
       3, 1-4.

338.   CHIAO, Y.-B., JOHNSTON, D.E., GAVALER, J.S., and VAN THIEL, D.H.
       (1981)   'Effect of chronic ethanol feeding on testicular
       content of enzymes required for testosteronogenesis.'   Alco-
       holism: Clinical and Experimental Research, 5, 230-236.

339. CHIAO, Y.-B., JOHNSTON, D.E., and VAN THIEL, D.H. (1980) 'Effect
      of chronic ethanol feeding on testicular content of enzymes
      required for testosteronogenesis.' Alcoholism: Clinical
      and Experimental Research, 4, 211 (abstract).

340. CHILDIAEVA, R., CHERNICK, V., and HAVLICEK, V. (1977) 'E.E.G.
      changes in infants of alcoholic mothers and infants of dia-
      betic mothers.' Proceedings of the International Union of
      Physiological Science, 13, 137.

341. CHOPRA, I.J., TULCHINSKY, D., and GREENWAY, F.L. (1973) 'Estro-
      gen-androgen imbalance in hepatic cirrhosis.' Annals of
      Internal Medicine, 79, 198-203.

342. CHRISTIAENS, L. (1961) 'La descendance des alcooliques.' ['The
      offspring of alcoholics.'] Annales de Pediatrie, 37, 380-
      381.

343. CHRISTIAENS, L., MIZON, J.P., and DELMARIE, G. (1960) 'Sur la
      descendance des alcooliques.' ['On the offspring of alco-
      holics.'] Annales de Pédiatrie, 36, 37-42.

344. CHRISTOFFEL, K.K., and SALAFSKY, I. (1975) 'Fetal alcohol syn-
      drome in dizygotic twins.' Journal of Pediatrics, 87, 963-
      967.

345. CHURCH, M.W., and HOLLOWAY, J.A. (1981) 'Audiogenic seizure
      susceptibility in mature rats with fetal alcohol syndrome.'
      Alcoholism: Clinical and Experimental Research, 5, 145 (ab-
      stract).

346. CHURCH, M.W., and HOLLOWAY, J.A. (1981) 'Brainstem auditory
      evoked response (Baer) in rats with fetal alcohol syndrome.'
      Alcoholism: Clinical and Experimental Research, 5, 145 (ab-
      stract).

347. CICERO, T.J. (1980) 'Sex differences in the effects of alcohol
      and other psychoactive drugs on endocrine function: Clin-
      ical and experimental evidence.' In: Research Advances in
      Alcohol and Drug Problems. Volume 5: Alcohol and Drug
      Problems in Women. Ed. O.J. Kalant. New York: Plenum
      Press, pp. 545-593.

348. CICERO, T.J., and BADGER, T.M. (1977) 'A comparative analysis
      of the effects of narcotics, alcohol and the barbiturates on
      the hypothalamic-pituitary-gonadal axis.' Advances in Ex-
      perimental Medicine and Biology, 85B, 95-115.

349. CICERO, T.J., and BADGER, T.M. (1977) 'Effects of alcohol on
      the hypothalamic-pituitary-gonadal axis in the male rat.'
      Journal of Pharmacology and Experimental Therapeutics, 201,
      427-433.

350. CICERO, T.J., and BELL, R.D.   (1979) Acetaldehyde directly in-
        hibits the conversion of androstenedione to testosterone in
        the testes.' Third International Symposium on Alcohol and
        Aldehyde Metabolizing Systems, p. 17 (abstract).

351. CICERO, T.J., and BELL, R.D.   (1980) 'Effects of ethanol and
        acetaldehyde on the biosynthesis of testosterone in the
        rodent testes.' Biochemical and Biophysical Research Com-
        munications, 94, 814-819.

352. CICERO, T.J., BELL, R.D., and BADGER, T.M. (1980) 'Acetaldehyde
        directly inhibits the conversion of androstenedione to tes-
        tosterone in the testes.' In: Alcohol and Acetaldehyde
        Metabolizing Systems-IV. (Advances in Experimental Medicine
        and Biology. Volume 132. Ed. R.G. Thurman. New York:
        Plenum Press, pp. 211-217.

353. CICERO, T.J., BELL, R.D., and BADGER, T.M. (1980) 'Multiple
        effects of ethanol on the hypothalamic-pituitary gonadal
        axis in the male.' In: Biological Effects of Alcohol: Pro-
        ceedings of the International Symposium on Biological Re-
        search in Alcoholism, Zurich, Switzerland (June, 1978).
        Ed. Henri Begleiter. New York: Plenum Press, pp. 463-478.

354. CICERO, T.J., BELL, R.D., MEYER, E.R., and BADGER, T.M. (1980)
        'Ethanol and acetaldehyde directly inhibit testicular
        steroidogenesis.' Journal of Pharmacology and Experimental
        Therapeutics, 213, 228-233.

355. CICERO, T.J., BERNSTEIN, D., and BADGER, T.M. (1978) 'Effects
        of acute alcohol administration on reproductive endocrinology
        in the male rat.' Alcoholism: Clinical and Experimental
        Research, 2, 249-254.

356. CICERO, T.J., MEYER, E.R., and BELL, R.D. (1979) 'Effects of
        ethanol on the hypothalamic-pituitary-luteinizing hormone
        axis and testicular steroidogenesis.' Journal of Pharmacol-
        ogy and Experimental Therapeutics, 208, 210-215.

357. CICERO, T.J., NEWMAN, K.S., and MEYER, E.R. (1980) 'Ethanol-
        induced inhibitions of testicular steroidogenesis in the
        male rat: Mechanisms of actions.' Life Sciences, 28, 871-
        877.

358. CLARK, R.A. (1952) 'The projective measurement of experimental-
        ly induced levels of sexual motivation.' Journal of Exper-
        imental Psychology, 44, 391-399.

359. CLARK, R.A., and SENSIBAR, M.R. (1955) 'The sexual relationship
        between symbolic and manifest projections of sexuality with
        some incidental correlates.' Journal of Abnormal and Social
        Psychology. 50, 327-334.

360. CLARREN, S.K. (1978) 'Central nervous system malformations in
        two offspring of alcoholic women.' Birth Defects, 13,
        151-153.

361. CLARREN, S.K.   (1979)   'Neural tube defects and fetal alcohol syn-
          drome.' [Letter.] Journal of Pediatrics, 98, 328.

362. CLARREN, S.K.   (1980)   'Alcohol vs. acetaldehyde as a teratogen.'
          Paper presented at the Fetal Alcohol Syndrome Workshop.
          Seattle, Washington (May 2-4).

363. CLARREN, S.K.   (1981)   'Recognition of fetal alcohol syndrome.'
          Journal of the American Medical Association, 245, 2436-2439.

364. CLARREN, S.K.   (1981)   'Summary and recommendations for clinical
          and dysmorphology studies of the fetal alcohol syndrome.'
          Neurobehavioral Toxicology and Teratology, 3, 239-240.

365. CLARREN, S.K., and ALVORD, E.C.   (1976)   'Leptomeingeal neuro-
          glial heterotopias in infants of alcoholic mothers.' Jour-
          nal of Neuropathology and Experimental Neurology, 35, 372.

366. CLARREN, S.K., ALVORD, E.C., SUMI, S.M., and STREISSGUTH, A.P.
          (1977)   'Brain malformation in offspring exposed to alcohol
          in utero.' Alcoholism: Clinical and Experimental Research,
          1, 159.

367. CLARREN, S.K., ALVORD, E.C., SUMI, S.M., STREISSGUTH, A.P., and
          SMITH, D.W.   (1978)   'Brain malformations related to prenatal
          exposure to ethanol.' Journal of Pediatrics, 92, 64-67.

368. CLARREN, S.K., and SMITH, D.W.   (1978)   'Fetal alcohol syndrome:
          Reply to letter to the editor.' New England Journal of Med-
          icine, 298, 556.

369. CLARREN, S.K., and SMITH, D.W.   (1978)   'The fetal alcohol syn-
          drome.' Lamp, 35, 4-7.

370. CLARREN, S.K., and SMITH, D.W.   (1978)   'The fetal alcohol syn-
          drome: A review of the world literature.' New England
          Journal of Medicine, 298, 1063-1067.

371. CLEGG, D.J.   (1964)   'The hen egg in toxicity and teratogenicity
          studies.' Food and Cosmetics Toxicology, 2, 717-727.

372. COBB, C.F., ENNIS, M.F., VAN THIEL, D.H., GAVALER, J.S., and LES-
          TER, R.   (1978)   'Acetaldehyde and ethanol are direct tes-
          ticular toxins.' Surgical Forum, 29, 641-644.

373. COBB, C.F., ENNIS, M.F., VAN THIEL, D.H., GAVALER, J.S., and LES-
          TER, R.   (1979)   'Alcohol: Its effect on the isolated per-
          fused rat testes.' Alcoholism: Clinical and Experimental
          Research, 3, 171 (abstract).

374. COBB, C.F., ENNIS, M.F., VAN THIEL, D.H., GAVALER, J.S., and LES-
          TER, R.   (1980)   'Isolated testes perfusion: A method using
          a cell- and protein-free perfusate useful for the evaluation
          of potential drug and/or metabolic injury.' Metabolism, 29,
          71-79.

375. COBO, E.   (1973)   'Effect of different doses of ethanol on the
     milk-ejecting reflex in lactating women.' American Journal
     of Obstetrics and Gynecology, 115, 817-821.

376. COBO, E., and QUINTERO, C.A. (1969) 'Milk-ejecting and anti-
     diuretic activities under neurohypophyseal inhibition with
     alcohol and water overload.' American Journal of Obstetrics
     and Gynecology, 105, 877-887.

377. COCCHI, M., MARZONA, L., PIGNATTI, C., and OLIVO, O.M. (1979)
     'Effects of ethanol on respiratory activity of embryonal tissues.'
     Bollettino Societa Italiana Biologica Speriment, 55, 423-426.

378. COHEN, M.M., JR. (1980) 'FAS and malignancies.' Paper pre-
     sented at the Fetal Alcohol Syndrome Workshop, Seattle,
     Washington (May 2-4).

379. COHEN, M.M., JR. (1981) 'Neoplasia and the fetal alcohol and
     hydantoin syndromes.' Neurobehavioral Toxicology and Tera-
     tology, 3, 161-162.

380. COLE, L.J., and BACKHUBER, L.J. (1914) 'The effect of lead on
     the germ cells of the male rabbit and fowl as indicated by
     their progeny.' Proceedings of the Society for Experimental
     Biology and Medicine, 12, 24.

381. COLE, L.J., and DAVIS, C.L. (1914) 'The effect of alcohol on
     the male germ cells, studied by means of double matings.'
     Science, 39, 476-477.

382. COLE, R., and COLE, J. (1976) 'Correlations between disturbed
     haem synthesis and fetal malformation.' Lancet (London), 2,
     640.

383. COLLARD, M.E., and CHEN, C.S. (1973) 'Effect of ethanol on
     growth of neonate mice as a function of modes of ethanol
     administration.' Quarterly Journal of Studies on Alcohol,
     34, 1323-1326.

384. COLLINS, E. (1980) 'Alcohol in pregnancy.' Medical Journal of
     Australia (Sydney), 2, 173-175.

385. COLLINS, E., and TURNER, G. (1978) 'Six children affected by
     maternal alcoholism.' Medical Journal of Australia (Syd-
     ney), 2, 606-608.

386. COMBEMALE, F. (1888) 'La descendance des alcooliques.' ['The
     offspring of alcoholics.'] Miscellaneous Nervous System,
     82, 14-213.

387. COMBES, J.C., BOSVIEUX, G., AUMERAS, C., PINSARD, N., and BER-
     NARD, R. (1980) 'Fetal alcohol syndrome.' Annals of
     Pediatrics, 27, 527-530.

388. CONNER, E.A., BLAKE, D.A., PARMLEY, T.H., BURNETT, L.S., and
      KING, T.M. (1976) 'Efficacy of various locally applied
      chemicals as contragestational agents in rats.' Contracep-
      tion, 13, 571-582.

389. COOK, L.N., SCHOTT, R.J., and ANDREWS, B.F. (1975) 'Acute
      transplacental ethanol intoxication.' American Journal of
      Diseases of Children, 129, 1075-1076.

390. COOK, P.S., ABRAMS, R.M., NOTELOVITZ, M., and FRISINGER, J.E.
      (1981) 'Effect of ethyl alcohol on maternal and fetal acid-
      base balance and cardiovascular status in chronic sheep
      preparations.' British Journal of Obstetrics and Gynecology,
      88, 188-194.

391. COOLEY-MATTHEWS, B., and TAYLOR, A.W. (1978) 'Exposure to eth-
      anol in utero may delay maturation of hypothalamo-pituitary
      adrenal function in the rat.' Neuroscience Abstracts (Ox-
      ford), 4, 318.

392. COOPER, P. (1978) 'Alcohol and the foetus.' Food and Cosmetics
      Toxicology (Oxford), 16, 290-292.

393. COOPER, P. (1980) 'Alcohol and pregnancy--Part 1: Animal
      data.' Food and Cosmetic Toxicology, 18, 312-314.

394. COOPER, S.J. (1978) 'Psychotropic drugs in pregnancy: Morpho-
      logical and psychological adverse effects on offspring.'
      Journal of Biosocial Science (London), 10, 321-334.

395. COOPERMAN, M.T., DAVIDOFF, F., SPARK, R., and PALLOTTA, J. (1974)
      'Clinical studies of alcoholic ketoacidosis.' Diabetes, 23,
      133-139.

396. COPPAGE, W.S., JR., and COONER, A.E. (1965) 'Testosterone in
      human plasma.' New England Medical Journal, 273, 902-907.

397. CORDES, H. (1898) 'Untersuchungen über den Einfluss acuter und
      chronischer Allgemeinerkrankungen auf die Testikel, special
      auf die Spermatogenese, sowie Beobachtungen über das Auf-
      treten von Fett in den Hoden.' ['Studies on the influence
      of acute and chronic general illnesses in the testicle,
      especially on spermatogenesis, as well as observations on
      the occurrence of fat in the testicle.'] Virchow's Archiv,
      151, 402.

398. CORRIGAN, G.E. (1976) 'The fetal alcohol syndrome.' Texas
      Medicine, 72, 72-74.

399. COTAESCU, I., DEUTSCH, G., and DREICHLINGER, O. (1965) 'The in-
      fluence of caffein, nicotine and ethanol on rat placentary
      blood circulation established by means of Rb^{86} uptake.'
      Revue Roumaine d'Embryologie et de Cytologie (Series D,
      Embryologie), 2, 31-35.

400. CRABBE, J.C., JANOWSKY, J.S., YOUNG, E.R., and RIGTER, H. (1980)
      'Strain-specific effects of ethanol on open field activity
      in inbred mice.' Substance Alcohol, Actions and Misuse, 1,
      537-543.

401. CRAWFORD, J.S. (1979) 'Premedication for elective Caesarean
      section.' Anaesthesia, 34, 892-897.

402. CROHOLM, J. (1968) 'Effect of ethanol on the concentrations of
      solvolyzable plasma steroids.' Biochimica et Biophysica
      Acta, 152, 233-236.

403. CRONHOLM, T., SJÖVALL, J., and SJÖVALL, K. (1969) 'Ethanol in-
      duced increase of the ratio between hydroxy and ketosteroids
      in human pregnancy plasma.' Steroids, 13, 671-678.

404. CROTHERS, T.D. (1887) 'Inebriety traced to the intoxication of
      parents at the time of conception.' Medical and Surgical
      Reporter, 56, 549-551.

405. CROWLEY, T.J., STYNES, A.J., HYDINGER, M. and KAUFMAN, I.C.
      (1974) 'Ethanol, methamphetamine, pentobarbital, morphine,
      and monkey social behavior.' Archives of General Psychiatry,
      31, 829-838.

406. CURLEE, J. (1969) 'Alcoholism and the "empty nest."' Bulletin
      of the Meninger Clinic, 33, 165.

407. CURRAN, F.J. (1937) 'Personality studies in alcoholic women.'
      Journal of Nervous and Mental Disease, 86, 645.

408. CUTLER, M.G. (1976) 'Changes in the social behavior of labora-
      tory mice during administration and on withdrawal from
      non-ataxic doses of ethyl alcohol.' Neuropharmacology
      (Oxford), 15, 495-498.

409. CUTLER, M.G., EWART, F.G., and MACKINTOSH, J.H. (1979) 'Growth
      and behavioural effects of ethyl alcohol on the offspring
      of mice; a comparison with its short-term actions.' Psycho-
      pharmacology, 66, 35-39.

410. CZAJKA, M.R., DANIELS, G., KAYE, G.I., and TUCCI, S.M. (1979)
      'Effects of ethanol on mouse embryos: Teratology and
      chromosome abnormalities.' Anatomical Record, 193, 515-516
      (abstract).

411. CZAJKA, M.R., TUCCI, S.M., and KAYE, G.I. (1980) 'Sister
      chromatid exchange frequency in mouse embryo chromosomes
      after in utero ethanol exposure.' Toxicology Letters, 6,
      257-261.

412. CZEIZEL, E. (1978) 'Az alkoholista nők terhességének epidemio-
      lógiai vizsgálata.' ['Epidemiological investigation of
      pregnancy among women alcoholics.'] Alkohológia (Budapest),
      9, 12-16.

D

413. DAHL, L.W. (1916) 'Über einige Resultate der Zählung der Geisteskranken in Norwegen den 31.' ['On a few results of the census of the mentally ill in Norway.'] Zeitschrift für Psychiatrie, 25, 839, 846.

414. DALBY, J.T. (1978) 'Environmental effects on prenatal development.' Journal of Pediatrics and Psychology, 3, 105-109.

415. DANFORTH, C.H. (1919) 'Evidence that germ cells are subject to selection on the bases of their genetic patient abilities.' Journal of Experimental Zoology, 28, 385-412.

416. DANIELS, M., and EVANS, M.A. (1980) 'Effect of maternal alcohol consumption on fetal and newborn development.' Federation Proceedings, 39 (Abstract #766).

417. DARBY, B.L. (1980) 'Prognostic implications of a birth diagnosis of FAS.' Paper presented at the Fetal Alcohol Syndrome Workshop, Seattle, Washington (May 2-4).

418. DARBY, B.L., STREISSGUTH, A.P., and SMITH, D.W. (1980) 'Prognostic implications of a fetal alcohol syndrome diagnosis in infancy.' Alcoholism: Clinical and Experimental Research, 4, 212 (abstract).

419. DARBY, B.L., STREISSGUTH, A.P., and SMITH, D.W. (1981) 'A preliminary follow-up of 8 children diagnosed fetal alcohol syndrome in infancy.' Neurobehavioral Toxicology and Teratology, 3, 157-159.

420. DA SILVA, V.A., LARANJEIRA, R.R., DOLNIKOFF, M., GRINFELD, H., and MASUR, J. (1981) 'Alcohol consumption during pregnancy and newborn outcome: A study in Brazil.' Neurobehavioral Toxicology and Teratology, 3, 169-172.

421. DA SILVA, V.A., MASUR, J., LARANJEIRA, R.R., DOLNIKOFF, M., and
      GRINFELD, H. (1980) 'Alcohol consumption during pregnancy
      by mothers of a low socioeconomical condition and their
      newborn.' Paper presented at the Fetal Alcohol Syndrome
      Workshop, Seattle, Washington (May 2-4).

422. DA SILVA, V.A., RIBEIRO, M.J., and MASUR, J. (1980) 'Develop-
      mental, behavioral, and pharmacological characteristics of
      rat offspring from mothers receiving ethanol during ges-
      tation and lactation.' Developmental Psychobiology, 13,
      653-660.

423. DAVENPORT, C.B. (1932) 'Effects of alcohol on animal off-
      spring.' In: Alcohol and Man. Ed. H. Emerson. New York:
      Macmillan, pp. 120-125.

424. DAVIDSON, S. (1981) 'Smoking and alcohol consumption: Advice
      given by health care professionals.' JOGN Nursing (Ju-
      ly/August), pp. 256-258.

425. DAVIDSON, S., ALDEN, L.E., and DAVIDSON, P.O. (1978) 'Changes
      in alcohol consumption after childbirth.' Paper presented
      at the XIX International Congress of Applied Psychology,
      Munich.

426. DAVIES, D.L., and SMITH, D.E. (1981) 'Effects of perinatally
      administered ethanol on hippocampal development.' Alco-
      holism: Clinical and Experimental Research, 5, 147 (ab-
      stract).

427. DAVIS, K. (1977) 'Alcohol linked to birth defects.' National
      Council on Alcoholism Reports (June 1), p. 1.

428. DAVIS, R. (1914) 'The effect of alcohol on the male germ cells,
      studied by means of double matings.' Science, New Series,
      39, 476-477.

429. DAVIS, V.E. (1980) 'The fetus and alcohol.' [Letter.] Medical
      Journal of Australia (Sydney), 1, 558.

430. DAY, S. (1980) 'Fetal alcohol syndrome.' Alcoholism: The
      National Magazine, 1, 35-36, 66.

431. DEBEUKELAER, M.M., and RANDALL, C.L. (1977) 'The fetal alcohol
      syndrome.' Journal of the South Carolina Medical Assoc-
      iation, 73, 407-412.

432. DEBEUKELAER, M.M., RANDALL, C.L., and STROUD, D.R. (1977)
      'Renal anomalies in the fetal alcohol syndrome.' Journal
      of Pediatrics, 91, 759-760.

433. DE CHÂTEAU, P. (1977) 'Ett fall av etylfetopati.' ['On the
      fetal alcohol syndrome.'] Läkartidningen (Stockholm), 72,
      1933.

434. DECKER, J.D., TUMBLESON, M.E., DEXTER, J.D., and MIDDLETON, C.
      (1980) 'Some teratogenic effects of ethanol on F-1 and F-2
      litters of miniature swine.' Anatomical Record, 196, 43a-
      44a (abstract).

435. DEHAENE, P.H., SAMAILLE-VILLETTE, C.H., SAMAILLE, P.-P., CRÉPIN,
      G., WALBAUM, R., DEROUBAIX, P., and BLANC-GARIN, A.P. (1977)
      'Le syndrome d'alcoolisme foetal dans le nord de la France.'
      ['The fetal alcohol syndrome in the north of France.']
      Revue de l'Alcoolisme (Paris), 23, 145-158.

436. DEHAENE, P.H., TITRAN, M., SAMAILLE-VILLETTE, C.H., SAMAILLE,
      P.-P., CRÉPIN, G., DELAHOUSSE, G., WALBAUM, R., and FAS-
      QUELLE, P. (1977) 'Fréquence du syndrome d'alcoolisme
      foetal.' ['Frequency of the fetal alcohol syndrome.']
      Nouvelle Presse Médicale (Paris), 6, 1703.

437. DEHAENE, P.H., WALBAUM, R., TITRAN, M., SAMAILLE-VILLETTE, C.H.,
      SAMAILLE, P.-P., CRÉPIN, G., DELAHOUSSE, G., DECOCQ, J.,
      DELCROIX, M., CAQUANT, F., and QUERLEU, D. (1977) 'La des-
      cendance des mères alcooliques chroniques. À propos de 16
      cas d'alcoolisme foetal.' ['Offspring of chronic alcoholic
      mothers. A report of 16 cases of fetal alcoholism.'] Revue
      Française de Gynécologie et d'Obstétrique, 72, 492-498.

438. DELGADO-RUBIO, A. (1980) 'Repercusiónes en el feto del alco-
      holismo crónico materno durante el embarazo.' ['The effects
      of chronic alcoholism on the fetus during pregnancy.'] In:
      Sociedad Cientifica Española sobre el Alcoholismo y las
      otras Toxicomanias. VII Jornadas Nacionales de Socidrogalco-
      hol, Pamplona, 27 al 29 de Septiembre de 1979. Ponencias y
      comunicaciónes. [The seventh National Meeting on Social
      Drugs and Alcohol, Pamplona (September 27-29). Papers and
      communications.] Pamplona.

439. DELPHIA, J.M., NEGULESCO, J.A., and FINAN, E. (1978) 'The ef-
      fect of ethanol on cerebral glycogen levels in the chick
      embryo.' Research Communications in Chemical Pathology and
      Pharmacology, 21, 347-350.

440. DE MEPEETERS, M. (1979) 'Impaired adaptation to extrauterine
      life: A teratogenic event.' In: Advances in the Study of
      Birth Defects. Volume 3: Abnormal Embryogenesis: Cellular
      and Molecular Aspects. Ed. T.V.N. Persaud. Baltimore,
      Maryland: University Park Press, pp. 193-218.

441. DEMERS, M., and KIROUAC, G. (1978) 'Prenatal effects of ethanol
      on the behavioral development of the rat.' Physiological
      Psychology, 6, 517-520.

442. DENDY, M. (1910) Letter on the notes made by Dr. Ashby con-
      cerning Manchester children and furnished to Elderton and
      Pearson. British Medical Journal (London), pp. 50-51, 348-
      349.

443. DENMARK, L.D. (1954) 'Smoking and drinking during pregnancy.'
       Journal of the American Medical Association, 154, 186.

444. DEPARTMENT OF HEALTH, EDUCATION, AND WELFARE. (1977) 'Fetal
       alcohol syndrome.' FDA Drug Bulletin, p. 18.

445. DEPARTMENT OF THE TREASURY, BUREAU OF ALCOHOL, TOBACCO, AND FIRE-
       ARMS. (1979) The Fetal Alcohol Syndrome: Public Awareness
       Campaign. Washington, D.C.: U.S. Government Printing
       Office.

446. DESESSO, J.M. (1979) 'Investigations into the modification of
       of hydroxy urea teratogenesis by the antioxidant propylgalatea.
       Anatomical Record, 193, 521 (abstract).

447. DETERING, N., COLLINS, R., HAWKINS, R., OZAND, P., and KARA-
       HASAN, A. (1980) 'Long lasting effects of prenatal ex-
       posure to ethanol in the rat.' Transactions of the American
       Society of Neurochemistry, 11, 246.

448. DETERING, N., COLLINS, R., OZAND, P.T., and KARAHASAN, A.M.
       (1979) 'The effects of ethanol (E) on developing catechol-
       amine neurons.' Third International Symposium on Alcohol
       and Aldehyde Metabolizing Systems, p. 24 (abstract).

449. DETERING, N., COLLINS, R., OZAND, P.T., and KARAHASAN, A.M.
       (1979) 'The effects of ethanol (E) on developing catechol-
       amine neurons.' Alcoholism: Clinical and Experimental Re-
       search, 3, 276 (abstract).

450. DETERING, N., EDWARDS, E., OZAND, P., and KARAHASAN, A.M. (1980)
       'Comparative effects of ethanol and malnutrition on the de-
       velopment of catecholamine neurons: Changes in specific
       activities of enzymes.' Journal of Neurochemistry, 34, 297-
       304.

451. DETERING, N., REED, W.P., OZAND, P.T., and KARAHASAN, A. (1979)
       'The effects of maternal ethanol consumption in the rat on
       the development of their offspring.' Journal of Nutrition,
       109, 999-1009.

452. DE TORCK, D. (1972) 'Chromosomal irregularities in alcoholics.'
       Annals of the New York Academy of Sciences, 197, 90-100.

453. DEWSBURY, D.A. (1967) 'Effects of alcohol ingestion on copula-
       tory behavior of male rats.' Psychopharmacologie (Berlin),
       11, 276-281.

454. DEXTER, J.D., and TUMBLESON, M.E. (1980) 'Fetal alcohol syn-
       drome in Sinclair (S-1) miniature swine.' Teratology, 21,
       35A-36A (abstract).

455.   DEXTER, J.D., TUMBLESON, M.E., DECKER, J.D., and MIDDLETON, C.C.
             (1979) 'Morphologic comparisons of piglets from first and
             second litters in chronic ethanol consuming Sinclair (S-1)
             miniature dams.' Alcoholism: Clinical and Experimental Re-
             search, 3, 171 (abstract). [Also in Pharmacology, Biochem-
             istry, and Behavior, 12, 324 (1980) as an abstract.]

456.   DEXTER, J.D., TUMBLESON, M.E., DECKER, J.D., and MIDDLETON, C.C.
             (1980) 'Fetal alcohol syndrome in Sinclair (S-1) miniature
             swine.' Alcoholism: Clinical and Experimental Research, 4,
             146-151.

457.   DEXTER, J.D., TUMBLESON, M.E., DECKER, J.D., and MIDDLETON, C.C.
             (1980) 'Morphologic comparison of piglets from first and
             second litters in chronic ethanol-consuming Sinclair (S-1)
             miniature swine.' In: Currents in Alcoholism. Volume 7:
             Recent Advances in Research and Treatment. Ed. M. Galanter.
             New York: Grune and Stratton, pp. 31-37.

458.   DEXTER, J.D., TUMBLESON, M.E., DECKER, J.D., and MIDDLETON, C.C.
             (1980) 'The comparison of the offspring of three serial
             pregnancies during voluntary alcohol consumption in Sinclair
             (S-1) miniature swine.' Alcoholism: Clinical and Exper-
             imental Research, 4, 213 (abstract).

459.   DEXTER, J.D., TUMBLESON, M.E., HUTCHESON, D.P., and MIDDLETON,
             C.C. (1976) 'Sinclair (S-1) miniature swine as model for
             the study of human alcoholism.' Annals of the New York
             Academy of Science, 273, 188-193.

460.   DIAZ, J., and SAMSON, H.H. (1980) 'Impaired brain growth in
             neonatal rats exposed to ethanol.' Science, 208, 751-753.

461.   DICKENS, G., and TRETHOWAN, W.H. (1971) 'Cravings and aversions
             during pregnancy.' Journal of Psychosomatic Research (Lon-
             don), 15, 259-268.

462.   DILTS, P.V., JR. (1970) 'Effect of ethanol on external and
             fetal umbilical hemodynamics and oxygen transfer.' American
             Journal of Obstetrics and Gynecology, 106, 221-228.

463.   DILTS, P.V., JR. (1970) 'Effect of ethanol on maternal and
             fetal acid-base balance.' American Journal of Obstetrics
             and Gynecology, 107, 1018-1021.

464.   DILTS, P.V., JR. (1970) 'Placental transfer of ethanol.'
             American Journal of Obstetrics and Gynecology, 107, 1195-
             1198.

465.   DIXIT, V.P., AGRAWAL, M., and LOHIYA, N.K. (1976) 'Effects of a
             single ethanol injection into the vas deferens on the tes-
             ticular function of rats.' Endokrinologie (Leipzig), 67,
             8-13.

466.   DOBBIE, J., and BILL, P. (1977) 'Fetal alcohol syndrome.' Ad-
             dictions (Toronto), 24, 5-15.

467. DOEPFMER, R., and HINCKERS, H.J. (1965) 'Zur Frage der Keim-
      schädigung im akuten Rausch.' ['On the question of germ-
      cell damage in acute alcohol intoxication.'] Zeitschrift
      für Haut und Geschlechtskrankheiten, 39, 94-107.

468. DOEPFMER, R., and HINCKERS, H.J. (1966) 'Zur Frage der Alkohol-
      einwirkung auf die Motilität menschlicher Spermien.' ['On
      the question of alcohol action on the mobility of human
      sperm.'] Zeitschrift für Haut und Geschlechtskrankheiten,
      40, 378-382.

469. DONATH, J. (1911) 'Die verebte Trunksucht mit besondere Rück-
      sicht auf die Dipsomainie.' ['The inherited addiction to
      drink with special attention to dipsomania.'] Öster-
      reichische Ärtzliche Vereins Zeitung (Vienna), 8, 18.

470. DOTSON, L.E., ROBERTSON, L.S., and TUCHFIELD, B. (1975) 'Plasma
      alcohol, smoking, hormone concentrations, and self-reported
      aggression.' Journal of Studies on Alcohol, 36, 578-586.

471. DREOSTI, I.E. (1981) 'Zinc deficiency and the fetal alcohol
      syndrome.' Medical Journal of Australia (Sydney), 2, 3-4.

472. DREOSTI, I.E., BALLARD, F.J., BELLING, G.B., RECORD, I.R.,
      MANUEL, S.J., and HETZEL, B.S. (1981) 'The effect of
      ethanol and acetaldehyde on DNA synthesis in growing cells
      and on fetal development in the rat.' Alcoholism: Clinical
      and Experimental Research, 5, 357-362.

473. DREOSTI, I.E., and RECORD, I.R. (1979) 'Superoxide dismutase
      (EC 1.15.1.1), zinc status and ethanol consumption in mater-
      nal and foetal rat livers.' British Journal of Nutrition,
      41, 399-402.

474. DRISCOLL, C.D., CHEN, J.S., and RILEY, E.P. (1980) 'Operant DRL
      and instrument runway performance in rats prenatally exposed
      to alcohol.' Paper presented at the Eastern Psychological
      Association, Hartford, Connecticut.

475. DRISCOLL, C.D., CHEN, J.S., and RILEY, E.P. (1980) 'Operant DRL
      performance in rats following prenatal alcohol exposure.'
      Neurobehavioral Toxicology, 2, 207-211.

476. DRISCOLL, C.D., CHEN, J.S., and RILEY, E.P. (1981) 'Passive
      avoidance performance in rats prenatally exposed to alcohol
      during various periods of gestation.' Neurobehavioral Tox-
      icology and Teratology (in press).

477. DRISCOLL, G.Z., and BARR, H.L. (1972) 'Comparative study of
      drug dependent and alcoholic women.' Selected papers of
      the 23rd Annual Meeting of the Alcohol and Drug Problems
      Association of North America, pp. 9-20.

478. DRUSE, M.J. (1980) 'Review of lipids and neurotransmitters.'
      Paper presented at the Fetal Alcohol Syndrome Workshop,
      Seattle, Washington (May 2-4).

479. DRUSE, M.J. (1981) 'Effects of maternal ethanol consumption on neurotransmitters and lipids in offspring.' Neurobehavioral Toxicology and Teratology, 3, 81-87.

480. DRUSE, M.J., and GNAEDINGER, J.M. (1980) 'Myelin-associated glycoproteins in the offspring of alcoholic rats.' Transactions of the American Society of Neurochemistry, 11, 153.

481. DRUSE, M.J., NORONHA, A.B., GNAEDINGER, J.M., and SMITH, D.M. (1980) 'Effects of maternal alcohol consumption and maternal malnutrition on CNS membranes in offspring.' Teratology, 21, 36A (abstract).

482. DRUSE-MANTEUFFEL, M.J., and HOFTEIG, J.H. (1977) 'The effect of chronic maternal alcohol consumption on the development of central nervous system myelin subfractions in rat offspring.' Drug and Alcohol Dependence (Lausanne), 2, 421-429.

483. DRUSE-MANTEUFFEL, M.J., and HOFTEIG, J.H. (1977) 'The effect of maternal alcohol consumption on the development and synthesis of three myelin subfractions in the rat.' Paper presented at the Milton Gross Memorial Symposium, Chicago.

484. DUMAS, R., and HADDAD, R. (1981) 'Teratogenicity of ethanol in the ferret.' Paper presented at the Conference on the Ferret as an Alternative Species in Teratology and Toxicology, Stanford, California (June 25-26).

485. DUMAS, R.M., and HADDAD, R.K. (1981) 'Teratogenicity of single doses of ethanol in CBA/J mice.' Teratology, 24, 53A (abstract).

486. DUMONT, M., THOULON, J.M., GUIBAND, S., BROUSSARD, P., and GLEHEN, D. (1977) 'Ethanol perfusions during threatened premature labor: Special study of oxytocinase activity.' Journal de Gynécologique, Obstétrique et Biologique de la Reproduction (Paris), 6, 107-116.

487. DUMONT, N. (1977) 'Hypotrophie foetale et intoxications maternelles chroniques.' ['Fetal hypotrophy and chronic maternal intoxication.'] Revue Française de Gynécologie et d'Obstétrique, 72, 797-803.

488. DUNCAN, R.J.S., and WOODHOUSE, B. (1978) 'The lack of effect on liver alcohol dehydrogenase in mice of early exposure to alcohol.' Biochemical Pharmacology, 27, 2755-2756.

489. DUNGAY, N.S. (1913) 'A study of the effects of injury upon the fertilizing power of sperm.' Biological Bulletin, 25, 213-216.

490. DUNMIRE-GRAFF, C.R. (1980) 'Effects of maternal ethanol consumption on developing facial motor neurons.' Anatomical Record, 196, 265.

491. DUNN, P.M., STEWART-BROWN, S., and PEEL, R. (1979) 'Metron-
      idazole and the fetal alcohol syndrome.' [Letter.] Lancet
      (London), 2, 144.

492. DUPUIS, C. (1979) 'Dangers de l'alcoolisme maternel; l'alcool,
      facteur de dysembryofoetopathie.' ['The dangers of maternal
      alcoholism; alcoholism as a factor in embryofetopathy.']
      Bulletin d'Information Alcoolisme, 139, 9-17.

493. DUPUIS, C. (1980) 'L'alcool, facteur de dysembryofoetopathie.'
      ['Alcohol, a factor of dysembryofetal pathology.'] Gazette
      Médicale de France, 87, 2539-2552.

494. DUPUIS, C., DEHAENE, P., DEROUBAIX-TELLA, P., BLANC-GARIN, A.P.,
      REY, C., and CARPENTIER-COURAULT, C. (1978) 'Les cardio-
      pathies des enfants nés de mère alcoolique.' ['Cardiac
      diseases in children born to alcoholic mothers.'] Archives
      des Maladies du Coeur et des Vaisseaux (Paris), 71, 565-572.

495. DURANDIN, R.M., and ROSSO, P. (1976) 'In vitro effects of eth-
      anol in human placental transport of amino acids.' Inter-
      national Research Communications System (IRES) Medical
      Science Library Compendium, 4, 439.

496. DURHAM, F.M., and WOODS, H.M. (1932) Alcohol and Inheritance:
      An Experimental Study. Great Britain Medical Research Coun-
      cil, Special Report Series, No. 168. London: H.M. Stat.,
      pp. 1-42.

497. DWORNIK, J.J., and MOORE, K.L. (1967) 'Congenital anomalies
      produced in the rat by podophyllin.' Anatomical Record,
      157, 237.

498. DYBAN, A.P., and KHOZHAĬ, L.I. (1980) 'Partenogeneticheskoye
      razvitiye ovulirovavshikh yaitsekletok mysheĭ pod vliyaniyem
      étilovogo spirta.' ['Parthenogenetic development of ovu-
      lated mouse ova induced by ethanol.'] Byulletin Eksper-
      imental'noi Biologii i Meditsiny, 89, 528-530.

E

501. EAGON, P.K., IMHOFF, A.F., and FISHER, S.E. (1978) 'Mechanism
     of hyperestrogenization in alcoholics: E_2/T ratio.'
     Twenty-ninth Annual Meeting of the American Association for
     the Study of Liver Disease, Chicago, Illinois.

502. EAGON, P.K., PORTER, L.E., GAVALER, J.S., EGLER, K.M., and
     VAN THIEL, D.H. (1981) 'Effect of ethanol feeding upon
     levels of a male-specific hepatic estrogen-binding protein:
     A possible mechanism for feminization.' Alcoholism: Clin-
     ical and Experimental Research, 5, 183-187.

503. EAST, W.N. (1932) 'Mental defectiveness and alcohol and drug
     addiction.' British Journal of Inebriety, 29, 149-168.

504. EDDY, C.C., and OLSON, C.M. (1980) 'Fetal alcohol syndrome and
     drinking during pregnancy.' In: Alcoholism in Women.
     Ed. C.C. Eddy and J.L. Ford. Dubuque, Iowa: Kendall/Hunt,
     pp. 109-116.

505. EDELSON, E. (1977) 'With child? Don't drink, group says.'
     National Council on Alcoholism Reports (June 19), p. 1.

506. EDITORIAL. (1976) 'Fetal alcohol syndrome.' Lancet (London),
     2, 1335.

507. EDITORIAL. (1976) 'The fetal alcohol syndrome.' British Med-
     ical Journal (London), 18, 1404-1405.

508. EDITORIAL. (1977) 'Pregnancy in the heavy drinker.' Lancet
     (London), 2, 647.

509. EDITORIAL. (1977) 'The fetal alcohol syndrome.' Alcoholism:
     Clinical and Experimental Research, 1, 191-192.

510. EDITORIAL. (1978) 'How important are genetic influences on al-
     cohol dependence?' British Medical Journal, 2, 1371-1372.

511. EDITORIAL. (1978) 'The fetal alcohol syndrome.' All Faith's
     World Alcohol Project Journal, 1, 51-53.

512. EDITORIAL. (1978) 'Warnings needed now.' All Faith's World
     Alcohol Project Journal, 1, 47-48.

513. EDUCATION COMMISSION OF THE STATES. (1980) 'What students
     should know about drinking and pregnancy.' [Brochure,
     10 pages.]

514. EHRLICH, W. (1910) 'La posterité des alcooliques.' ['The off-
     spring of alcoholics.'] Thèse, Lausanne.

515. ELDERTON, E., and PEARSON, K. (1910) 'A first study of the in-
     fluence of parental alcoholism on the physique and ability of
     the offspring.' Eugenics Laboratory Memoirs, 10, 46-57.

516. EL-GUEBALY, N., and OFFORD, D.R. (1977) 'The offspring of alco-
     holics: A critical review.' American Journal of Psychiatry,
     134, 357-365.

517. EL-GUEBALY, N., and OFFORD, D.R. (1979) 'On being the offspring
     of an alcoholic: An update.' Alcoholism: Clinical and Ex-
     perimental Research, 3, 148-157.

518. ELIS, J. (1979) 'Effect of drugs applied during pregnancy on
     postnatal development.' Evaluation of Embryotoxic, Muta-
     genic, and Carcinogenic Risks of New Drugs, pp. 141-144.

519. ELIS, J., and KRŠIAK, M. (1975) 'Effect of alcohol adminis-
     tration during pregnancy on social behaviour of offspring
     in mice.' Activitas Nervosa Superior (Prague), 17, 281-282.

520. ELIS, J., KRŠIAK, M., and PÖSCHLOVÁ, N. (1978) 'Effect of alco-
     hol given at different periods of gestation on brain sero-
     tonin in offspring.' Activitas Nervosa Superior (Prague),
     20, 287-288.

521. ELIS, J., KRŠIAK, M., PÖSCHLOVÁ, N., and MASEK, K. (1976) 'The
     effect of alcohol administration during pregnancy on concen-
     tration of noradrenaline, dopamine and 5-hydroxytryptamine
     in the brain of offspring of mice.' Activitas Nervosa
     Superior (Prague), 18, 220-221.

522. ELLINGBOE, J., MENDELSON, J.H., KUEHNLE, J.C., SKUPNY, A.S.T.,
     and MILLER, K.D. (1980) 'Effect of acute ethanol ingestion
     on integrated plasma prolactin levels in normal men.' Phar-
     macology, Biochemistry, and Behavior, 12, 297-301.

523. ELLINGBOE, J., and VARANELLI, C.C. (1979) 'Ethanol inhibits
     testosterone biosynthesis by direct action on Leydig cells.'
     Research Communications in Chemical Pathology and Pharma-
     cology, 24, 87-102.

524. ELLIS, F.W. (1980) 'Effects of short term exposure in Beagle
     dogs.' Paper presented at the Fetal Alcohol Syndrome Work-
     shop, Seattle, Washington (May 2-4).

525. ELLIS, F.W., and PICK, J.R.   (1976)   'Beagle model of the fetal
      alcohol syndrome.'   Pharmacologist, 18, 190 (abstract).

526. ELLIS, F.W., and PICK, J.R.   (1979)   'Fetal exposure to ethanol
      during short segments of gestation.'   Pharmacologist, 21,
      188 (abstract #232).

527. ELLIS, F.W., and PICK, J.R.   (1980)   'An animal model of the
      fetal alcohol syndrome in beagles.'   Alcoholism: Clinical
      and Experimental Research, 4, 123-134.

528. ELLIS, F.W., and PICK, J.R.   (1981)   'A beagle model of the fetal
      alcohol syndrome.'   British Journal on Alcohol and Alco-
      holism, 16, 47-49.

529. ELLIS, F.W., PICK, J.R., and SAWYER, M.   (1977)   'Effects of
      ethanol administration during pregnancy on fetal development
      in beagle dogs.'   Federation Proceedings, 36, 285.

530. ELLIS, F.W., PICK, J.R., and SAWYER, M.   (1977)   'Ethanol dose-
      response relationships in a beagle model of the fetal alco-
      hol syndrome.'   Paper presented at the Fetal Alcohol Syn-
      drome Workshop, San Diego, California.

531. ELTON, R.H., and WILSON, M.E.   (1977)   'Changes in ethanol con-
      sumption by pregnant pigtailed macaques.'   Journal of
      Studies on Alcohol, 38, 2181-2183.

532. EMERSON, G.A., BROWN, R.G., NASH, J.B., and MOORE, W.T.   (1952)
      'Species variation in preference for alcohol and in effects
      of diet or drugs on this preference.'   Journal of Pharmacol-
      ogy and Experimental Therapeutics, 106, 384 (abstract).

533. ENOS, W.F., and BEYER, J.C.   (1980)   'Prostatic acid phosphatase,
      aspermia, and alcoholism in rape cases.'   Journal of Foren-
      sic Science, 25, 353-356.

534. ERB, L., and ANDRESEN, B.D.   (1978)   'The fetal alcohol syndrome
      (F.A.S.): A review of the impact of chronic maternal alco-
      holism in the developing fetus.'   Clinical Pediatrics, 17,
      644-649.

535. ERIKSSON, K.   (1979)   'Alkoholinkäyttö ja perintötekijät.'
      ['Drinking behavior and genetics.']   Duodecim, 95, 347-356.

536. ERIKSSON, M., LARSSON, G., and ZETTERSTRÖM, R.   (1979)   'Abuse of
      alcohol, drugs, and tobacco during pregnancy--Consequences
      for the child.'   Paediatrician, 8, 228-242.

537. ESKAY, R.L., RYBACK, R.S., GOLDMAN, M., and MAJCHROWICZ, E.
      (1981)   'Effect of chronic ethanol administration on plasma
      levels of LH and the estrous cycle in the female rat.'   Al-
      coholism: Clinical and Experimental Research, 5, 204-206.

538. ESKES, T.K. (1979) 'Het foetale alcoholsyndroom.' ['The fetal alcohol syndrome.'] Nederlands Tijdschrift voor Geneeskunde, 123, 1276-1279.

539. ETZIONI, A. (1977) 'Caution: Too many health warnings could be counterproductive.' Psychology Today, pp. 20-22.

540. ETZIONI, A. (1979) 'A systematic and graduated response.' In: The Fetal Alcohol Syndrome: Public Awareness Campaign. The Department of the Treasury and The Bureau of Alcohol, Tobacco, and Firearms. Washington, D.C.: U.S. Government Printing Office.

541. EUNICE KENNEDY SHRIVER CENTER FOR MENTAL RETARDATION, INC. (1980) 'Alcohol and pregnancy.' [Brochure.]

542. EUNICE KENNEDY SHRIVER CENTER FOR MENTAL RETARDATION, INC. (1980) 'Teenagers and alcohol.' [Brochure.]

543. EUNICE KENNEDY SHRIVER CENTER FOR MENTAL RETARDATION, INC. (1980) 'What you should know about alcohol and your baby.' [Brochure.]

544. EVANS, A.N.W., BROOKE, O.G., and WEST, R.J. (1980) 'The ingestion by pregnant women of substances toxic to the foetus.' Practitioner, 224, 315-319.

545. EWART, F.G., and CUTLER, M.G. (1979) 'Effects of ethyl alcohol on behaviour in nursing female mice.' Psychopharmacology (Berlin), 66, 143-146.

546. EWART, F.G., and CUTLER, M.G. (1979) 'Effects of ethyl alcohol on development and social behaviour in offspring of laboratory mice.' Psychopharmacology (Berlin), 62, 247-251.

547. EWING, J.A. (1968) 'Alcohol, sex, and marriage.' Medical Aspects of Human Sexuality, 4, 43-50.

548. EZCURDIA, M. (1980) 'Alcohol y embarazo.' ['Alcohol and pregnancy.'] In: Sociedad Cientifica Espagnola sobre el Alcoholismo y las otras Toxicomanias; VII Jornadas Nacionales de Socidrogalcohol, Pamplona, 27 al 29 de Septiembre de 1979: Ponencias y comunicacio/alnes. [The VII National Meeting on Social Drugs and Alcohol, Pamplona, 27-29 September, 1979: Papers and Communications.] Pamplona, pp. 145-150.

F

549. FABRE, L.F., PASCO, P.J., LIEGEL, J.M., and FARMER, R.W. (1973) 'Abnormal testosterone excretion in men alcoholics.' Quarterly Journal of Studies on Alcoholism, 34, 57-63.

550. FABRO, SERGIO E. (1979) 'Alcoholic beverage consumption and outcome of pregnancy.' In: The Fetal Alcohol Syndrome: Public Awareness Campaign. The Department of the Treasury and The Bureau of Alcohol, Tobacco, and Firearms. Washington, D.C.: U.S. Government Printing Office.

551. FAHIM, M.S., DEMENT, G., and HALL, D.G. (1970) 'Induced alterations in hepatic metabolism of androgens in the rat.' American Journal of Obstetrics and Gynecology, 107, 1085-1091.

552. FARKAS, G.M., and ROSEN, R.C. (1976) 'Effect of alcohol on elicited male sexual response.' Journal of Studies on Alcohol, 37, 265-272.

553. FARNSWORTH, W.E., CAVANAUGH, A.H., BROWN, J.R., ALVAREZ, I., and LEWANDOWSKI, L.M. (1978) 'Factors underlying infertility in the alcoholic.' Archives of Andrology, 1, 193-195.

554. FARRELL, J.I. (1938) 'The secretion of alcohol by the genital tract: An experimental study.' Journal of Urology, 40, 62-65.

555. FARRY, K., and TITTMAR, H.-G. (1975) 'Alcohol as a teratogen: Effects of maternal administration in rats on sexual development in female offspring.' Pharmacology, Reproduction, Obstetrics and Gynecology, 3, 619-620.

556. FEIFER, MAXINE. (1979) 'Don't Start Your Baby on the Drink.' Forum, 12.

557. FENDER, F., and STREISSGUTH, A.P. (1980) 'What physicians tell their patients about drinking and smoking during pregnancy: A pilot study.' Unpublished report.

558. FERE, C.H. (1893) 'Note sur l'influence de l'exposition preal-
      able aux vapeurs d'alcool sur l'incubation de l'oeuf de la
      poule.' ['Note on the influence of preliminary exposure to
      the vapors of alcohol on the incubation of the egg of the
      hen.'] Comptes Rendus des Seances de la Société de Biologie
      et de ses Filiales (Paris), pp. 773-775.

559. FERE, C.H. (1894) 'Action teratogene de l'alcool methylique.'
      ['Teratogenic action of methyl alcohol.'] Comptes Rendus
      des Seances de la Société de Biologie et de ses Filiales
      (Paris), p. 221.

560. FERE, C.H. (1894) 'Poulets vivants provenant d'oeufs ayant subi
      des injections d'alcool ethylique dans l'albumen.' ['Live
      chickens lay eggs having undergone injections of ethyl
      alcohol in the albumen.'] Comptes Rendus des Seances de
      la Société de Biologie et de ses Filiales (Paris), p. 646.

561. FERE, C.H. (1894) 'Presentation de poulets vivants provenant
      d'oeufs ayant subi des injections d'alcool ethylique dans
      l'albumen.' ['Presentation of living chicks from eggs which
      had undergone ethanol injections in the albumen.'] Comptes
      Rendus des Seances de la Société de Biologie et de ses
      Filiales (Paris), 46, 646.

562. FERE, C. H. (1895) 'Etudes experimentales sur l'influence tera-
      togene ou degénérative des alcools et des essences.' ['Ex-
      perimental studies on the teratogenic or degenerative influ-
      ence of alcohol and its essences.'] Journal de l'Anatomie
      et de la Physiologie, 31, 161-186.

563. FERE, C. H. (1899) 'Influence de repos sur les effets de l'ex-
      position prealable aux vapeurs de l'alcool avant l'incuba-
      tion, etc.' ['Influence of sleep on the effects of pre-
      liminary exposure to alcoholic vapors before incubation,
      etc.'] Comptes Rendus des Seances de la Société de Biologie
      et de ses Filiales (Paris), p. 225.

564. FERNANDEZ, K., CAUL, W.F., BOYD, J.E., HENDERSON, G.I., and
      MICHAELIS, R.C. (1980) 'Teratogenic effects of prenatal
      ethanol exposure as a function of gestational age?' Paper
      presented at the International Society for Developmental
      Psychobiology, Cincinnati, Ohio (November 8).

565. FERNANDEZ, K., CAUL, W.F., and MARSEE, H.G. (1981) 'Increased
      activity in young rats prenatally exposed to ethanol.'
      Teratology, 24, 54A (abstract).

566. FERNANDEZ, K., CAUL, W.F., OSBORNE, G.L., and HENDERSON, G.I.
      (1979) 'Effect of maternal chronic ethanol administration
      on offspring, open field, and Y maze performance.' Paper
      presented at the International Society for Developmental
      Psychobiology, Atlanta, Georgia (November).

567. FERRIER, P.E.   (1979) 'L'embryopathie alcoholique.' ['Fetal
      alcohol syndrome' (editorial).] Helvetica Paediatrica Acta
      (Basel), 34, 105-106.

568. FERRIER, P.E.   (1979) 'Le syndrome de l'alcoolisme foetal:
      "Fetal alcohol syndrome."' ['The fetal alcohol syndrome.']
      Bulletin der Schweizerischen Akademie der Medizinischen
      Wissenschaften, 35, 147-150.

569. FERRIER, P.E., NICOD, I., and FERRIER, S. (1973) 'Fetal alcohol
      syndrome.' [Letter.] Lancet (London), 2, 1496.

570. FETAL ALCOHOL SYNDROME. (1976) Film produced by the National
      Broadcasting Company. Landers Film Reviews (September/Octo-
      ber), 21, 13.

571. FETCHKO, A.M., WEBER, J.E., CARROLL, J.H., and THOMAS, G.J.
      (1951) 'Intravenous alcohol used for preinduction analgesia
      in obstetrics.' American Journal of Obstetrics and Gynecol-
      ogy, 62, 662-664.

572. FICHER, M., and LEVITT, D.R. (1980) 'Testicular dysfunction and
      sexual impotence in the alcoholic rat.' Journal of Steroid
      Biochemistry, 13, 1089-1095.

573. FIELDING, J., and YANKAUER, A. (1978) 'The pregnant drinker.'
      American Journal of Public Health, 68, 836-838.

574. FIGA-TALAMANCA, I., and MODOLO, M.A. (1977) 'A study of behav-
      ioral aspects of infant mortality in an Italian community.'
      International Journal of Health Education (Geneva), 20, 248-
      258.

575. FIGUERIDO, C.A. (1947) 'Los ilamados males germinales y los des-
      cendientes de toxicomanos.' ['So-called germ damage and the
      offspring of addicts.'] Revista de Sanidad Higiene Publica
      (Madrid), 21, 1215-1221.

576. FINNEGAN, L. (1980) 'Interactions between drugs and hazards to
      pregnancy.' Focus on Alcohol and Drug Issues, 3, 14-15.

577. FINNEGAN, L.P. (1981) 'The effects of narcotics and alcohol on
      pregnancy and the newborn.' Annals of the New York Academy
      of Sciences, 362, 136-157.

578. FINUCANE, B.T. (1980) 'Difficult intubation associated with the
      foetal alcohol syndrome.' Canadian Anaesthesiology Society
      Journal, 27, 574-575.

579. FIOCCHI, A., COLOMBINI, A., and CODARA, L. (1978) 'La embrio-
      patia alcoolica; rassegna della letteratura e contributo
      personale.' ['Alcohol embryopathy; literature review and
      personal contribution.'] Minerva Paediatrica (Torino), 30,
      19-28.

580. FISH, B.S., RANK, S.H., WILSON, J.R., and COLLINS, A.C. (1980)
'Viability and sensorimotor development of mice exposed to
prenatal short-term ethanol.' Pharmacology, Biochemistry,
and Behavior, 14, 57-65.

581. FISHER, M., and LEVITT, D.R. (1978) 'Effects of alcohol on rat
testicular steroidogenesis.' Sixtieth Annual Meeting--Endo-
crinology Society, Miami, Florida.

582. FISHER, S.E., ATKINSON, M.B., HOLZMAN, I.R., DAVID, R., and VAN
THIEL, D.H. (1981) 'Ethanol-associated inhibition of human
placental amino acid uptake: A new concept in the fetal
alcohol syndrome (FAS).' Alcoholism: Clinical and Experimental Research, 5, 149 (abstract).

583. FISHER, S.E., ATKINSON, M., HOLZMAN, I., and VAN THIEL, D.H.
(1981) 'In vitro inhibition of human placental amino acid
(A-A) uptake: Synergism between nicotine (Nic) and acetaldehyde (AcH).' Alcoholism: Clinical and Experimental Research, 5, 149 (abstract).

584. FISHER, S.E., BARNICLE, M.A., STEIS, B., and HOLZMAN, I. (1979)
'Fetal alcohol syndrome diminished in utero swallowing and
intestinal uptake of amino-acid by the fetal rat.' Gastroenterology, 76, 1133.

585. FISHER, S.E., BARNICLE, M.A., STEIS, B., HOLZMAN, I., and VAN
THIEL, D.H. (1980) 'Acute ethanol exposure and protein
synthesis in the fetal rat: Dose-response.' Alcoholism:
Clinical and Experimental Research, 4, 214 (abstract).

586. FISHER, S.E., BARNICLE, M.A., STEISS, B., HOLZMAN, I., and VAN
THIEL, D.II. (1981) 'Effects of acute ethanol exposure upon
in vivo leucine uptake and protein synthesis in the fetal
rat.' Pediatric Research, 15, 335-339.

587. FITZE, F., SPAHR, A., and PESCIA, G. (1978) 'Familienstudie zum
Problem des embryofötalen Alkoholsyndroms.' ['Fetal alcohol
syndrome: Follow-up of a family.'] Schweizerische Rund-
schau Medizin (PRAXIS), 67, 1338-1354.

588. FLEIT, L. (1979) Alcohol and Sexuality: A Handbook for the
Counselor/Therapist. Arlington, Virginia: H/P Publishing
Company.

589. FLETCHER, J.M., COWAN, E.A., and ARLITT, A.H. (1916) 'Experiments on the behavior of chicks hatched from alcoholized
eggs.' Journal of Animal Behavior, 6, 103-137.

590. FLYNN, A., MILLER, S.I., and DEL VILLANO, B.C. (1980) 'Maternal
and newborn blood zinc as an indicator for alcohol related
fetal defects.' Drug and Alcohol Dependence, 6, 45-46.

591. FLYNN, A., MILLER, S.I., MARTIER, S.S., GOLDEN, N.I., SOKOL,
      R.J., and DEL VILLANO, B.C. (1981) 'Zinc status of preg-
      nant alcoholic women: A determinant of fetal outcome.'
      Lancet (London), 1, 572.

592. FOREL, A. (1893) 'The effect of alcoholic intoxication upon the
      human brain and its relation to the theories of heredity and
      evolution.' Quarterly Journal of Inebriety, 12, 203-221.

593. FOREL, A. (1911) 'Alkohol und keim Zellen (Blastophthorische
      Entartung).' ['Alcohol and developing cells (blastophthoric
      degeneration).'] Münchener Medizinische Wochenschrift
      (Munich), 49, 2596.

594. FOX, H.E., STEINBRECHER, M., PESSEL, D., INGLIS, J., MEDVID, L.,
      and ANGEL, E. (1978) 'Maternal ethanol ingestion and the
      occurrence of human fetal breathing movements.' American
      Journal of Obstetrics and Gynecology, 132, 354-358.

595. FRANK, L.M., and ROSMAN, N.P. (1978) 'Studies on growth,
      learning, and morphogenesis in experimental fetal alcohol
      syndrome.' Annals of Neurology, 4, 195-196.

596. FREEMAN, C. (1975) 'Preliminary human trial of a new male ster-
      ilization procedure: Vas sclerosing.' Fertility and Ster-
      ility, 26, 162-166.

597. FREEMAN, C., and COFFEY, D.S. (1973) 'Male sterility induced
      by ethanol injection into the vas deferens.' International
      Journal of Fertility, 18, 129-132.

598. FREEMAN, C. and COFFEY, D.S. (1973) 'Sterility in male animals
      induced by injection of chemical agents into the vas defer-
      ens.' Fertility and Sterility, 24, 884-890.

599. FRETS, G.P. (1931) Alcohol and the Other Germ Poisons. Nij-
      hoff: The Hague.

600. FRICKER, H.S. and SEGAL, S. (1978) 'Narcotic addiction, preg-
      nancy and the newborn.' American Journal of Diseases in
      Children, 132, 360-366.

601. FRIEBEL, D. (1979) 'Beitrag zur Alkohol-Embryopathie.' ['Alco-
      hol embryopathy.'] Kinderärztliche Praxis, 47, 584-590.

602. FRIED, P.A., WATKINSON, B., GRANT, A., and KNIGHTS, R.M. (1980)
      'Changing patterns of soft drug use prior to and during
      pregnancy: A prospective study.' Drug and Alcohol Depen-
      dence, 6, 323-343.

603. FRIED, R.I., and RAVIN, J.G. (1978) 'Fetal alcohol syndrome.'
      Journal of Pediatric Ophthalmology and Strabismus, 15, 394-
      395.

604.   FRISCO, B.   (1909)   'Influenza perturbatrice dell'alcool sul plasma germinativo ed creditarieta morbose dei discendenti consecutive all'alcoolismo dei genitori.'   ['Disturbing influence of alcohol on the germinative plasma and morbidity of consecutive descendants of alcoholic parents.']   Annali Della Clinica delle Malattie Mentali e Nervose della Reale Universita di Palermo, 3, 383-435.

605.   FRITCHIE, G.E., HO, B.T., and MC ISAAC, W.M.   (1972)   'Autoradiographic study of ^{14}C-ethanol: Incorporation of ^{14}C-ethanol and metabolites in monkey brain and fetus.'   In: Biological Aspects of Alcohol.   Ed. M.K. Roach, W.M. Mc Isaac, and P.J. Creaven.   Austin, Texas, and London: University of Texas Press, pp. 285-292.

606.   FRYNS, J.P., DEROOVER, J., PARLOIR, C., GOFFAUX, P., LEBAS, E., and VAN DEN BERGHE, H.   (1977)   'The foetal alcohol syndrome.'   Acta Paediatrica Belgica (Brussels), 30, 117-121.

607.   FUCHS, A.-R.   (1964)   'Oxytocin and the onset of labour in rabbits.'   Journal of Endocrinology (London), 30, 217-224.

608.   FUCHS, A.-R.   (1966)   'The inhibitory effect of ethanol on the release of oxytocin during parturition in the rabbit.'   Journal of Endocrinology (London), 35, 125-134.

609.   FUCHS, A.-R.   (1969)   'Ethanol and the inhibition of oxytocin release in lactating rats.'   Acta Endocrinologica (Copenhagen), 62, 546-554.

610.   FUCHS, A.-R.   (1978)   'Hormonal control of myometrial function during pregnancy and parturition.'   Acta Endocrinologica (Copenhagen), Supplement No. 221, 1-70.

611.   FUCHS, A.-R., and WAGNER, G.   (1963)   'Effect of alcohol on release of oxytocin.'   Nature, 198, 92-94.

612.   FUCHS, A.-R., and WAGNER, G.   (1963)   'The effect of ethyl alcohol on the release of oxytocin in rabbits.'   Acta Endocrinologica (Copenhagen), 44, 593-605.

613.   FUCHS, F.   (1976)   'Treatment of imminent premature labour.'   [Letter.]   Acta Obstetrica et Gynecologica Scandinavica (Lund), 55, 379.

614.   FUCHS, F.   (1981)   'Ethanol and premature infants--reply.'   American Journal of Obstetrics and Gynecology, 140, 351.

615.   FUCHS, F., FUCHS, A.-R., LAUERSEN, N.H., and ZERVOUDAKIS, I.A.   (1979)   'Treatment of pre-term labor with ethanol.'   Danish Medical Bulletin, 26, 123-124.

616.   FUCHS, F., FUCHS, A.-R., POBLETE, V.F., JR., and RISK, A.   (1967)   'Effect of alcohol on threatened premature labor.'   American Journal of Obstetrics and Gynecology, 99, 627-637.

617.   FUCHS, M., IOSUB, S., BINGOL, N., and GROMISCH, D.S.   (1980)
       'Palpebral fissure size revisited.'   Journal of Pediatrics,
       96, 77-78.

618.   FUEYO-SILVA, A., MENÉNDEZ-PATTERSON, A., and MARIN, B.   (1980)
       'Efectos del consumo prenatal del alcohol sobre la fecundidad,
       natalidad, crecimiento, apertura vaginal y ciclo sexual en la
       rata.'   ['Effects of prenatal alcohol consumption upon fecun-
       dity, natality, growth, vaginal opening, and sexual cycle in
       the rat.']   Reproduccion, 4, 265-270.

619.   FUKUDA, Y., and TOYODA, Y.   (1974)   'Effects of oral administration
       of ethanol on ovulation and embryonic development in the rat.'
       Japanese Journal of Fertility and Sterility, 19, 46-52.

620.   FURNAS, J.C.   (1965)   The Life and Times of the Late Demon Rum.
       New York: Capricorn Books.

621.   FUSTER, J.S., GUELL, S., CAHUANA, A.B., and GARCIATORNEL, S.
       (1979)   'Neural tube defects with fetal alcohol syndrome.'
       [Letter.]   Journal of Pediatrics, 95, 328.

G

622. GABRIEL, E. (1934) 'Nie Nachkommenschaft von Alkoholikern.' Archiv für Psychiatrische Nervenkrankheiten, 102, 506-537.

623. GALLANT, D.M. (1968) 'The effect of alcohol and drug abuse on sexual behavior.' Medical Aspects of Human Sexuality, 2, 30-36.

624. GALLANT, D.M. (1981) 'Similarities between the fetal alcohol syndrome and phenylketonuria anomalies.' Alcoholism: Clinical and Experimental Research, 5, 575.

625. GALLO, P.V., and WEINBERG, J. (1981) 'Prenatal alcohol exposure: Neuromotor development and postweaning response inhibition.' Teratology, 24, 54A (abstract).

626. GALVÃO-TELES, A., ANDERSON, D.C., BURKE, C.W., and MARSHALL, J.C. (1973) 'Biologically active androgens and oestradiol in men with chronic liver disease.' Lancet (London), 1, 173-177.

627. GANTT, W.H. (1952) 'Effect of alcohol in the sexual reflexes of normal and neurotic male dogs.' Psychosomatic Medicine, 14, 174-181.

628. GARCÍA-TAMAYO, J., ROJAS, T., VOEGLER, M.I., SIBLESZ, M.I., CASTRO, C., and MOROS, M.A. (1980) 'Purkinje cell alterations in newborn rats after maternal administration of ethanol: Light and electron microscopy.' Paper presented at the Post-Congress Meeting of the International Academy of Pathology, Budapest (September).

629. GARDNER, R.J.M., and CLARKSON, J.E. (1981) 'A malformed child whose previously alcoholic mother had taken disulfiram.' New Zealand Medical Journal, 93, 184-186.

630. GARRIDO-LESTACHE, J. (1976) 'La madre, et alcohol y la descendencia.' ['Mother, alcohol and offspring.'] Anales de la Real Academica Nacional de Medicina (Madrid), 93, 495-505.

631. GARTNER, U., and RYDEN, G.   (1972)   'The elimination of alcohol in the premature infant.' Acta Paediatrica Scandinavica (Stockholm), 61, 720-721.

632. GAVALER, J.S., VAN THIEL, D.H., and LESTER, R.   (1980)   'Ethanol: A gonadal toxin in the mature rat of both sexes.' Alcoholism: Clinical and Experimental Research, 4, 271-276.

633. GEBHART, E.   (1979)   'Zur Frage der erbgutschädigenden Nebenwirkungen von psychotropen Substanzen. Teil 2: Rausch- und Suchtdrogen.' ['Mutagenic effects of psychotropic substances. Part 2. Narcotics and addictive drugs.'] Fortschritte der Medizin, 97, 103-106.

634. GEE, W.   (1916)   'Effects of acute alcoholization on the germ cells of fundulus heteroclitus.' Biological Bulletin, 31, 297-406.

635. GHISHAN, F.K., HENDERSON, G., and MENEELY, R.   (1981)   'Intestinal function in infant rats: Effect of maternal chronic ethanol ingestion.' Journal of Nutrition, 3, 1124.

636. GIARETTO, G., BINI, P., JARRE, L., and BASILE, F.   (1979)   'Malformazioni morfologiche cerebrali e renali in sospetta sindrome alcoolica fetale: Contributo clinico.' ['A case of cerebral and renal morphological deformities in a patient with suspected foetal alcoholic syndrome: Clinical contribution.'] Minerva Pediatrica, 31, 1185-1190.

637. GIBBENS, G.L.D., and CHARD, T.   (1976)   'Observations on maternal oxytocin release during human labor and the effect of intravenous alcohol administration.' American Journal of Obstetrics and Gynecology, 126, 243-246.

638. GIESE, A.C.   (1948)   'Effects of alcohol on fertilization in the sand dollar.' Anatomical Record, 101, 709-710.

639. GIKNIS, M.L.A., and DAMJANOV, I.   (1980)   'The teratogenetic and embryotoxic effects of alcohol in four mouse strains.' Teratology, 21, 40A (abstract).

640. GIKNIS, M.L.A., DAMJANOV, I., and RUBIN, E.   (1980)   'The differential transplacental effects of ethanol in four mouse strains.' Neurobehavioral Toxicology, 2, 235-237.

641. GILBEAU, P.M., SMITH, C.G., and BESCH, N.F.   (1981)   'Comparison of the acute effects of marijuana, ethanol, and morphine on sex hormone levels in the male rhesus monkey.' Journal of Andrology, 2, 13 (abstract).

642. GILDER, S.S.B.   (1974)   'Alcohol, tobacco and pregnancy.' Canadian Medical Association Journal (Toronto), 110, 903.

643. GILFORD, H.   (1912)   'Alcoholism and problems of growth and development.' British Journal of Inebriety, 9, 173-179.

644. GILMAN, M.R.   (1971) 'A preliminary study of the teratogenic ef-
      fects of inhaled carbon tetrachloride and ethyl alcohol con-
      sumption in the rat.' Dissertation Abstracts, 32, 2021.

645. GIMENO, M.A.F., BEDNERS, A.S., DE VASTIK, F.J., and GIMENO, A.L.
      (1971) 'Effect of ethanol on motility of isolated rat myometrium.
      Archives internationales Pharmacodnamie Thérapie, 191, 213-219.

646. GINSBURG, B.E., YANAI, J., and HEDRICK, B. (1977) 'Nutritionally
      mediated effects of alcohol administered to pregnant and
      lactating mice on the behavior of their offspring.' Behavior
      Genetics, 7, 61-62 (abstract).

647. GINSBURG, B.E., YANAI, J., and SZE, P.Y. (1975) 'A developmenta-
      genetic study of the effects of alcohol consumed by parent
      mice on the behavior and development of their offspring.'
      NIAAA Proceedings of the 4th Annual Alcoholism Conference of
      the National Institute on Alcohol Abuse and Alcoholism, 1974.
      The Institute: Rockville, Maryland, pp. 183-204.

648. GLOOR, P.A. (1952) 'Alcoolisme et selection.' ['Alcoholism and
      selection.'] Schweizer Archiv für Neurologie und Psych-
      iatrie, 70, 445-453.

649. GNANAPRAKASAM, M.S., CHEN, C.J.H., SUTHERLAND, J.G., and BHALLA,
      V.K. (1979) 'Receptor depletion and replenishment pro-
      cesses: In vivo regulation of gonadotropin receptors by
      luteinizing hormone, follicle stimulating hormone and eth-
      anol in rat testis.' Biological Reproduction, 20, 991-1000.

650. GOAD, P.T., HILL, D.E., SLIKKER, W., JR., KIMMEL, C.A., and GAY-
      LOR, D.W. (1981) 'The developmental effects of ethanol and
      the role of maternal nutrition.' Teratology, 24, 54A (ab-
      stract).

651. GOAD, P.T., SLIKKER, W., JR., KIMMEL, C.A., GAYLOR, D.W., and
      HILL, D.E. (1980) 'Maternal and fetal toxicity of ethanol:
      Role of altered nutrition.' Clinical Research, 28, 872a.

652. GODLEWSKI, J. (1980) 'Problematyka alkoholowa w seksuologii.'
      ['Alcohol problems in sexology.'] Problemy Alkoholizmu
      (Warsaw), 27, 7-8.

653. GOETZMAN, B.W., KAGAN, J., and BLANKENSHIP, W.J. (1975) 'Expan-
      sion of the fetal alcohol syndrome.' Clinical Research, 23,
      100.

654. GOLDSTEIN, G., and ARULANANTHAM, K. (1978) 'Neural tube defect
      and renal anomalies in a child with fetal alcohol syndrome.'
      Journal of Pediatrics, 93, 636-637.

655. GOMEL, V., and CARPENTER, C.W. (1973) 'Induction of midtrimes-
      ter abortion with intrauterine alcohol.' Journal of Obstet-
      rics and Gynecology, 41, 455-458.

656. GONZÁLEZ, E.R.   (1981)   'New ophthalmic findings in fetal alcohol syndrome.' Journal of the American Medical Association, 245, 108.

657. GORDIS, E., and KREEK, M.J.   (1977)   'Alcoholism and drug addiction in pregnancy.' In: Current Problems in Obstetrics and Gynecology. Volume I: Alcoholism and Drug Addiction in Pregnancy. Chicago: Year Book Medical Publishers, pp. 1-48.

658. GORDON, A.   (1911)   'Parental alcoholism as a factor in the mental deficiency of children; a statistical study of 117 families.' Journal of Inebriety, 33, 90-99.

659. GORDON, A.   (1913)   'A study of fourteen cases of alcoholism in children apparently free from morbid heredity.' Medical Record, 33, 423-435.

660. GORDON, A.   (1913)   'Parental alcoholism as a factor in the mental deficiency of children; a statistical study of 117 families.' Journal of Inebriety, 35, 58-65.

661. GORDON, A.   (1916)   'The influence of alcohol on the progeniture.' International Medical Journal, 23, 431-436.

662. GORDON, B.H.J., STREETER, , and WINICK, M.   (1981)   'Placental development in alcohol fed rats.' Federation Proceedings, 40, 799 (abstract).

663. GORDON, G.G., ALTMAN, K., SOUTHREN, A.L., RUBIN, E., and LIEBER, C.S.   (1976)   'Effect of alcohol (ethanol) administration on sex-hormone metabolism in normal men.' New England Journal of Medicine, 295, 793-797.

664. GORDON, G.G., and LIEBER, C.S.   (1979)   'The fetal alcohol syndrome: Mechanisms and models.' [Editorial.] Hospital Practice, 14, 11, 15.

665. GORDON, G.G., OLIVO, J., RAFIN, F., and SOUTHREN, A.L.   (1975)   'Conversion of androgens to estrogens in cirrhosis of the liver.' Journal of Clinical Endocrinology and Metabolism, 40, 1018-1026.

666. GORDON, G.G., SOUTHREN, A.L., and LIEBER, C.S.   (1978)   'The effects of alcoholic liver disease and alcohol ingestion on sex hormone levels.' Alcoholism: Clinical and Experimental Research, 2, 259-263.

667. GORDON, G.G., SOUTHREN, A.L., and LIEBER, C.S.   (1979)   'Hypogonadism and feminization in the male: A triple effect of alcohol.' [Editorial.] Alcoholism: Clinical and Experimental Research, 3, 210-212.

668. GORDON, G.G., VITTEK, J., HO, R., ROSENTHAL, W.S., SOUTHREN, A.L., and LIEBER, C.S.   (1979)   'Effect of chronic alcohol use on hepatic testosterone 5-α-A-ring reductase in the baboon and in the human being.' Gastroenterology, 77, 11-114.

669. GORDON, G.G., VITTEK, J., SOUTHREN, A.L., MUNNANGI, P., and
      LIEBER, C.S. (1980) 'Effect of chronic alcohol ingestion
      on the biosynthesis of steroids in rat testicular homogenate
      in vitro.' Endocrinology, 106, 1880-1885.

670. GORDON, G.G., VITTEK, J., WEINSTEIN, B., SOUTHREN, A.L., and
      LIEBER, C.S. (1979) 'Acute and chronic effects of alcohol
      on steroid hormones with emphasis on the metabolism of andro-
      gens and estrogens.' In: Metabolic Effects of Alcohol:
      Proceedings of the International Symposium on Metabolic
      Effects of Alcohol, Milan (June 18-21). Ed. P. Avogaro,
      C.R. Sirtori, and E. Tremoli. New York: Elsevier, pp. 89-
      102.

671. GORDON, G.G., WORNER, T.M., SOUTHREN, A.L., and LIEBER, C.S.
      (1981) 'Abnormal gonadotrophin releasing hormone responses
      in chronically alcoholic men.' Alcoholism: Clinical and
      Experimental Research, 5, 151 (abstract).

672. GORDON, N. (1978) 'Fetal drug syndromes.' Postgraduate Medical
      Journal, 54, 796-798.

673. GOUJARD, J., KAMINSKI, M., RUMEAU-ROUQUETTE, C., and SCHWARTZ, D.
      (1978) 'Maternal smoking, alcohol consumption, and abruptio
      placentae.' [Letter.] American Journal of Obstetrics and
      Gynecology, 130, 738-739.

674. GRAFF, G. (1971) 'Failure to prevent premature labor with eth-
      anol.' American Journal of Obstetrics and Gynecology, 110,
      878-880.

675. GRAHAM, J.M., JR., DARBY, B.L., BARR, H.M., SMITH, D.W., and
      STREISSGUTH, A.P. (1981) 'Long-term effects of alcoholic
      consumption during pregnancy.' Teratology, 23, 38A (ab-
      stract).

676. GRAHAM, J.M., JR., DARBY, B.L., BARR, H.M., SMITH, D.W., and
      STREISSGUTH, A.P. (1981) 'Long-term effects of moderate
      alcohol consumption during pregnancy.' Pediatric Research,
      15, 643 (abstract #1203).

677. GRANT, K., SAMSON, H.H., and DIAZ, J. (1981) 't-butanol induced
      microcephaly in the neonatal rat.' Alcoholism: Clinical
      and Experimental Research, 5, 151 (abstract).

678. GRAUWILER, J., LEIST, K.H., and SCHOEN, H. (1975) 'A test for
      behavior of young rats in teratological experiments.' Tera-
      tology, 12, 329-330 (abstract).

679. GRAY, S.L., POTTS, F.L., and MEANS, L.W. (1981) 'Failure of
      neonatal ethanol exposure to impair maze acquisition in
      rats.' International Research Communication System: Med-
      ical Science Library Compendium, 9, 16.

680. GREEN, H.G.   (1974)   'Infants of alcoholic mothers.' American
          Journal of Obstetrics and Gynecology, 118, 713-716.

681. GREEN, J.R., MOWAT, N.A., and FISHER, R.A.   (1976)   'Plasma estro-
          gens in men with chronic liver disease.' Gut (London), 17,
          426-430.

682. GREEN, V.A.   (1970)   'Effects of pesticides on rat and chick em-
          bryo.' Trace Substances and Environmental Health--3, Pro-
          ceedings of the University of Missouri, Third Annual Confer-
          ence, pp. 183-209.

683. GREENE, L.W., and HOLLANDER, C.S.   (1980)   'Sex and alcohol: The
          effects of alcohol on the hypothalamic-pituitary-gonadal
          axis.' [Guest editorial.] Alcoholism: Clinical and Exper-
          imental Research, 4, 1-5.

684. GREENHOUSE, B.S., HOOK, R., and HEHRE, F.W.   (1969)   'Aspiration
          pneumonia following intravenous administration of alcohol
          during labor.' Journal of the American Medical Association,
          210, 168-171.

685. GREIZERSTEIN, H.B., and ABEL, E.L.   (1979)   'Acute effects of
          ethanol on fetal body composition and electrolyte content in
          the rat.' Bulletin of the Psychonomic Society, 14, 355-356.

686. GREIZERSTEIN, H.B., and ABEL, E.L.   (1980)   'Time parameters for
          increased blood ethanol disappearance rates in lactating
          rats.' Alcoholism: Clinical and Experimental Research, 4,
          216 (abstract).

687. GREIZERSTEIN, H.B., ABEL, E.L., and SIEMENS, A.J.   (1979)   'Lac-
          tation and ethanol disappearance in the rat.' Pharmacol-
          ogist, 21, 188 (abstract #233).

688. GRENIER, L.   (1887)   'Contribution à l'étude de la descendance
          des alcooliques.' ['Contribution to the study of the off-
          spring of the alcoholic.'] Thèse, Paris.

689. GUNEV, V.   (1980)   'Fetalen alkokholen sindrom.' ['Fetal alcohol
          syndrome.'] Akusherstvo i Ginekologiya (Sofia), 19, 66-70.

690. GUZINSKI, G.M., LITTLE, R.E., and STREISSGUTH, A.P.   (1979)   'Con-
          sequences of alcohol use in pregnancy: A summary.' King
          County Medical Society Bulletin, 58, 19.

H

691. HABBICK, B.F., ZALESKI, W.A., CASEY, R., and MURPHY, F. (1979) 'Liver abnormalities in three patients with fetal alcohol syndrome.' Lancet (London), 1, 580-581.

692. HADDAD, R., CANLON, B., DUMAS, R., LEE, M., and RABE, A. (1979) 'Maternal ethanol consumption during pregnancy affects fetal skeletal development in the rat.' Paper presented at the Laboratory Animal Science Meeting, Atlanta, Georgia (October).

693. HADDON, J. (1876) 'On intemperance in women, with special reference to its effects on the reproductive system.' British Medical Journal (London), 1, 748-750.

694. HAGBERG, B., HAGBERG, G., LEWERTH, A., and LINDBERG, U. (1981) 'Mild mental retardation in Swedish school children. II. Etiologic and pathogenetic aspects.' Acta Paediatrica Scandinavica, 70, 445-452.

695. HAGGARD, H.W., and JELLINEK, E.M. (1942) Alcohol Explored. Garden City: Doubleday.

696. HALKKA, O., and ERIKSSON, K. (1977) 'The effects of chronic ethanol consumption on goniomitosis in the rat.' In: Alcohol Intoxication and Withdrawal. Volume 3A. Ed. Milton M. Gross. New York: Plenum Publishing Corporation, pp. 1-6.

697. HALL, B.D., and ORENSTEIN, W.A. (1974) 'Noonan's phenotype in an offspring of an alcoholic mother.' [Letter.] Lancet (London), 1, 680-681.

698. HALL, J.G. (1979) Letter to the Bureau of Alcohol, Tobacco and Firearms. In: The Fetal Alcohol Syndrome: Public Awareness Campaign. The Department of the Treasury and The Bureau of Alcohol, Tobacco and Firearms. Washington, D.C.: U.S. Government Printing Office.

699. HAMMER, R.P., JR., and SCHEIBEL, A.B. (1981) 'Morphologic evi-
      dence for a delay of neuronal maturation in fetal alcohol
      exposure.' Experimental Neurology (in press).

700. HAMMOND, D.C., JORGENSEN, G.Q., and RIDGEWAY, D.M. (1980)
      'Sexual adjustment of female alcoholics.' Medical Aspects
      of Human Sexuality (in press).

701. HANSON, F.B. (1927) 'Do Albino rats having ten generations of
      alcoholic ancestry inherit resistance to alcohol fumes?'
      American Naturalist, 59, 53.

702. HANSON, F.B. (1932) 'Modifications in the Albino rat following
      treatment with alcohol fumes and x-rays; and the problem of
      their inheritance.' Proceedings of the American Philosoph-
      ical Society, 62, 301-310.

703. HANSON, F.B., and COOPER, Z.K. (1930) 'The effects of ten gener-
      ations of alcoholic ancestry upon learning ability in the Al-
      bino rat.' Journal of Experimental Zoology, 56, 369-392.

704. HANSON, F.B., and HANDY, V. (1923) 'The effects of alcohol fumes
      on the albino rat: Introduction and sterility data for the
      first treated generation.' American Naturalist, 57, 532-544.

705. HANSON, F.B., and HEYS, F. (1924) 'Correlations of body weight,
      body length, and tail length in normal and alcoholic albino
      rats.' Genetics, 9, 368-371.

706. HANSON, F.B., and HEYS, F. (1925) 'Alcohol and the sex ratio.'
      Genetics, 10, 351-358.

707. HANSON, F.B., and HEYS, F. (1927) 'Alcohol and eye defects in
      the albino rat.' Journal of Heredity, 18, 345.

708. HANSON, F.B., and HEYS, F. (1927) 'Do albino rats having ten
      generations of alcoholic ancestry inherit resistance to al-
      cohol fumes?' American Naturalist, 61, 43-53.

709. HANSON, F.B., and HEYS, F. (1927) 'The effects of alcohol on
      birthweight and litter size in the albino rat.' American
      Naturalist, 61, 503.

710. HANSON, F.B., SHOLES, F.N., and HEYES, F. (1928) 'Alcohol and
      body weight in the albino rat.' Genetics, 13, 121-125.

711. HANSON, J.W. (1977) 'Alcohol and the fetus.' British Journal
      of Hospital Medicine (London), 18, 128-130.

712. HANSON, J.W., JONES, K.L., and SMITH, D.W. (1976) 'Fetal alco-
      hol syndrome: Experience with 41 patients.' Journal of the
      American Medical Association, 235, 1458-1460.

713. HANSON, J.W., JONES, K.L., and SMITH, D.W. (1976) 'The fetal
      alcohol syndrome.' Journal of the American Medical Assoc-
      iation, 236, 1114.

714. HANSON, J.W., STREISSGUTH, A.P., and SMITH, D.W. (1978) 'The ef-
           fects of moderate alcohol consumption during pregnancy on
           fetal growth and morphogenesis.' Journal of Pediatrics, 92,
           457-460.

715. HARKONEN, M., SEUDERLING, U., ONIKKI, S., KARONEN, S.-L., and
           ADLER-CREUTZ, H. (1974) 'Low plasma testosterone values in
           men during hangover.' Journal of Steroid Biochemistry (Ox-
           ford), 5, 655-658.

716. HARLAP, S. (1980) 'Moderate alcohol use and spontaneous abor-
           tions: A prospective study.' Papers presented by P.H. Shi-
           ono at the Fetal Alcohol Syndrome Workshop, Seattle, Washing-
           ton (May 2-4).

717. HARLAP, S., and SHIONO, P.H. (1980) 'Alcohol, smoking, and in-
           cidence of spontaneous abortions in the first and second tri-
           mester.' Lancet, 2, 173-176.

718. HARLAP, S., SHIONO, P.H., and RAMCHARAN, S. (1979) 'Alcohol and
           spontaneous abortions.' American Journal of Epidemiology,
           110, 372 (abstract).

719. HARLAP, S., SHIONO, P.H., and RAMCHARAN, S. (1979) 'Alcohol,
           smoking and the incidence of spontaneous first and second
           trimester abortions.' Unpublished manuscript. Kaiser-
           Permanente Birth Defects Study, Kaiser-Permanente Medical
           Center, Walnut Creek, California.

720. HARLAP, S., SHIONO, P.H., RAMCHARAN, S., BERENDES, H., and PEL-
           LEGRIN, F. (1979) 'A prospective study of spontaneous
           fetal losses after induced abortions.' New England Journal
           of Medicine, 301, 677-681.

721. HARRIES, J.M., and HUGHES, T.F. (1958) 'Enumeration of the
           "cravings" of some pregnant women.' British Medical Journal
           (London), 2, 35-40.

722. HARRIS, J.M., and PASHAYAN, H.M. (1976) 'Teratogenesis.' Ortho-
           pedic Clinics of North America, 7, 281-289.

723. HARRIS, R.A., and CHASE, J. (1979) 'Effects of maternal consump-
           tion of ethanol, barbital, or chlordiazepoxide on the behaviour
           of offspring.' Behavioral and Neural Biology, 26, 234-247.

724. HARRIS, R.A., and CHASE, J. (1978) 'Maternal consumption of
           ethanol, barbital or chlordiazepoxide: Effects on behaviour
           of the offspring.' Neuroscience Abstracts (Oxford), 4, 493.

725. HART, B.L. (1968) 'Effects of alcohol on sexual reflexes and
           mating behavior in the male dog.' Quarterly Journal of Studies
           on Alcohol, 29, 839-844.

726. HART, B.L. (1969) 'Effects of alcohol on sexual reflexes and
           mating behavior in the male rat.' Psychopharmacologia (Ber-
           lin), 14, 377-382.

727. HASSAN, M.M., and LONGMORE, D.B. (1973) 'Effects of contracep-
      tive pill constituents on fetal mouse hearts.' Nature (Lon-
      don), 244, 349-351.

728. HAUGHTON, G., MOHR, K., and ELLIS, F. (1981) 'Increased
      susceptibility to induction of primary Rous sarcoma in
      C57BL/10ScSn mice following perinatal exposure to dietary
      ethanol.' Alcoholism: Clinical and Experimental Research,
      5, 347 (abstract).

729. HAUSCHILD, R., SEEWALD, H.-J., and ZORN, C. (1973) 'Die pharma-
      kologische Beeinflussung der Aktivität des menschlichen Myo-
      metriums im in-vitro-Versuch. III. Äthanol-Wirkung auf das
      isolierte Uterusmuskelsstreifenpreparat.' ['Pharmalogical
      modification of human myometrium activity in studies in
      vitro. III. Effect of ethanol on isolated myometrial strip
      preparations.'] Zentralblatt für Gynäkologie (Leipzig), 95,
      769-771.

730. HAVERS, W., MAJEWSKI, F., OLBING, H., and EICKENBERG, H.-U.
      (1980) 'Anomalies of the kidneys and genitourinary tract in
      alcohol embryopathy.' Journal of Urology, 124, 108-110.

731. HAVLICEK, V., and CHILDIAEVA, R. (1976) 'EEG component of fetal
      alcohol syndrome.' Lancet (London), 2, 477.

732. HAVLICEK, V., and CHILDIAEVA, R. (1981) 'Sleep EEG in newborns
      of mothers using alcohol.' In: Fetal Alcohol Syndrome.
      Volume 2: Human Studies. Ed. E.L. Abel. Boca Raton, Flor-
      ida: CRC Press (in press).

733. HAVLICEK, V., CHILDIAEVA, R., and CHERNICK, V. (1975) 'EEG fre-
      quency spectrum characteristics of sleep states in full-term
      and preterm infants.' Neuropädiatrie, 6, 24.

734. HAVLICEK, V., CHILDIAEVA, R., and CHERNICK, V. (1977) 'EEG fre-
      quency spectrum characteristics of sleep rates in infants of
      alcoholic mothers.' Neuropädiatrie, 8, 360-373.

735. HAWKINS, D.F. (1976) 'Teratogens in the human: Current prob-
      lems.' Journal of Clinical Pathology, 29 (Supplement 10),
      150-156.

736. HAWKINS, J.L. (1976) 'Lesbianism and alcoholism.' In: Alco-
      holism Problems in Women and Children. Ed. M. Greenblatt
      and M.A. Schuckit. New York: Grune and Stratton, pp. 137-
      141.

737. HAYDEN, M.R., and NELSON, M.M. (1978) 'The fetal alcohol syn-
      drome.' South African Medical Journal (Cape Town), 54, 571-
      574.

738. HEALTH CAUTION IN FETAL ALCOHOL SYNDROME. (1977) U.S. Depart-
      ment of Health, Education, and Welfare (June).

739. HEALY, P. (1980) 'The pregnant cause campaign: An explanation
      and an outline.' Focus Women, 1, 204-213.

740. HEARLE, J.M. (1980) 'Conference on fetal alcohol syndrome.'
      Quality Review Bulletin, 6, 24-29.

741. HEMMINKI, E., and STARFIELD, B. (1978) 'Prevention and treatment
      of premature labour by drugs: Review of controlled clinical
      trials.' British Journal of Obstetrics and Gynecology (Lon-
      don), 85, 411-417.

742. HENDERSON, G.I. (1980) 'Effects of ethanol on placental func-
      tion.' Paper presented at the Fetal Alcohol Syndrome Work-
      shop, Seattle, Washington (May 2-4).

743. HENDERSON, G.I., HOYUMPA, A.M., JR., MC CLAIN, C., and SCHENKER,
      S. (1979) 'The effects of chronic and acute alcohol admin-
      istration on fetal development in the rat.' Alcoholism:
      Clinical and Experimental Research, 3, 99-106.

744. HENDERSON, G.I., HOYUMPA, A., PATWARDHAN, R., and SCHENKER, S.
      (1981) 'Effect of acute and chronic ethanol exposure on pla-
      cental uptake of amino acids.' Alcoholism: Clinical and Ex-
      perimental Research, 5, 153 (abstract).

745. HENDERSON, G.I., HOYUMPA, A.M., JR., ROTHSCHILD, M.A., and SCHEN-
      KER, S. (1980) 'Effect of ethanol and ethanol-induced hypo-
      thermia on protein synthesis in pregnant and fetal rats.'
      Alcoholism: Clinical and Experimental Research, 4, 165-177.

746. HENDERSON, G.I., HOYUMPA, A.M., JR., and SCHENKER, S. (1979)
      'Role of ethanol-induced hypothermia on net protein syn-
      thesis (NPS) in maternal and fetal tissues.' Third Inter-
      national Symposium on Alcohol and Acetaldehyde Metabolizing
      Systems, p. 16 (abstract).

747. HENDERSON, G.I., PATWARDHAN, R.V., HOYUMPA, A.M., JR., and SCHEN-
      KER, S. (1981) 'Fetal alcohol syndrome: Overview of path-
      ogenesis.' Neurobehavioral Toxicology and Teratology, 3,
      73-80.

748. HENDERSON, G.I., and SCHENKER, S. (1977) 'The effects of mater-
      nal alcohol consumption on the viability and visceral devel-
      opment of the newborn rat.' Research Communications in
      Chemical Pathology and Pharmacology, 16, 15-32.

749. HENDERSON, G.I., and SCHENKER, S. (1981) 'The inhibition of
      fetal growth by maternal ethanol consumption--Two potential
      mechanisms.' Teratology, 23, 40A-41A (abstract).

750. HENDERSON, G.I., TURNER, D., PATWARDHAN, R.V., LUMENG, L.,
      HOYUMPA, A.M., and SCHENKER, S. (1981) 'Inhibition of
      placental valine uptake after acute and chronic maternal
      ethanol consumption.' Journal of Pharmacology and Exper-
      imental Therapeutics, 216, 465-472.

751. HERMAN, C.S., KIRCHNER, G.L., STREISSGUTH, A.P., and LITTLE, R.E.
      (1980) 'Vigilance paradigm for preschool children used to
      relate vigilance behavior to IQ and prenatal exposure to al-
      cohol.' Perceptual and Motor Skills, 50, 863-867.

752. HERMAN, C.S., LITTLE, R.E., STREISSGUTH, A.P., and BECK, D.E.
      (1980) 'Alcoholic fathering and its relation to child's in-
      tellectual development.' Alcoholism: Clinical and Exper-
      imental Research, 4, 217 (abstract).

753. HERMIER, M., LECLERCQ, F., DUC, H., DAVID, L., and FRANÇOIS, R.
      (1976) 'Le nanisme intra-utérin avec débilité mentale et
      malformations dans le cadre de l'embryofoetopathie alcool-
      ique; à propos de quatre cas.' ['Intrauterine growth defic-
      iency with mental retardation and malformations in alcoholic
      embryo-fetopathy; concerning four cases.'] Pédiatrie
      (Lyons), 31, 749-762.

754. HERRMANN, J., PALLISTER, P.D., and OPITZ, J.M. (1980) 'Tetra-
      ectrodactyly and other skeletal manifestations in the fetal
      alcohol syndrome.' European Journal of Pediatrics, 133, 221-
      226.

755. HEUYER, H., MISES, R., and DEREUX, J.F. (1957) 'La descendance
      des alcooliques.' ['The offspring of alcoholics.'] Presse
      Médicale (Paris), 29, 657-658.

756. HILL, D.E., SLIKKER, W., JR., GOAD, P.T., BAILEY, J.R., and HEN-
      DRICKX, A.G. (1981) 'Transplacental pharmacokinetics of
      ethanol in rhesus and cynomolgus monkeys.' Teratology, 23,
      41A (abstract).

757. HILL, L.G., DANIN, S.T., and MEANS, L.W. (1981) 'Alcohol con-
      sumption during gestation and maternal behavior in the rat.'
      Alcoholism: Clinical and Experimental Research, 5, 350 (ab-
      stract).

758. HILL, R.M. (1976) 'Fetal malformations and antiepileptic
      drugs.' American Journal of Diseases of Children, 130,
      923-925.

759. HILL, R.M., CRAIG, J.P., CHANEY, M.D., TENNYSON, L.M., and MC CUL-
      LEY, L.B. (1977) 'Utilization of over-the-counter drugs
      during pregnancy.' Clinical Obstetrics and Gynecology, 20,
      381-394.

760. HILL, R.M., and HORNING, M.G. (1974) 'Effect on the infant of
      drug therapy of the mother.' Current Topics in Clinical
      Chemistry, 2, 103-112.

761. HILL, R.M., and TENNYSON, L.M. (1980) 'An historical review and
      longitudinal study of an infant with the fetal alcohol syn-
      drome.' In: Alcoholism: A Perspective. Ed. F.S. Messiha
      and G.S. Tyner. Westbury, New York: PJD Publications,
      pp. 177-201.

762. HIMWICH, W.A., HALL, J.S., and MAC ARTHUR, W.F. (1977) 'Maternal alcohol and neonatal health.' Biological Psychiatry, 12, 495-505.

763. HINCKERS, H.J. (1976) 'Alcohol and pregnancy: Negative and positive effects of acute and chronic action of alcohol on the course and outcome of pregnancy.' [In German.] Fortschritte der Medizin, 94, 1771-1782.

764. HINCKERS, H.J. (1978) 'The influences of alcohol on the fetus.' Journal of Perinatal Medicine (Berlin), 6, 3-14.

765. HO, B.T., FRITCHIE, G.E., IDÄNPÄÄN-HEIKKILÄ, J.E., and MC ISAAC, W.M. (1972) 'Placental transfer and tissue distribution of ethanol-1-^{14}C: A radioautographic study in monkeys and hamsters.' Quarterly Journal of Studies on Alcohol, 33, 485-493.

766. HODGE, C.F. (1903) 'The influence of alcohol on growth and development.' In: Physiological Aspects of the Liquor Problem. Volume I. Ed. W.O. Atwater, J.S. Billings, H.P. Bowditch, R.H. Chittenden, and W.H. Welch. Boston: Houghton-Mifflin, pp. 359-375.

767. HOENNICKE, A. (1907) 'Über experimentale erzeugte Missbildungen.' ['On experimentally created defects.'] Münchener Medizinische Wochenschrift (Munich), 54, 2065.

768. HOFTEIG, J.H., and DRUSE-MANTEUFFEL, M.J. (1978) 'Central nervous system myelination in rats exposed to ethanol in utero.' Drug and Alcohol Dependence (Lausanne), 3, 429-434.

769. HOFTEIG, J.H., DRUSE-MANTEUFFEL, M.J., and COLLINS, M.A. (1976) 'The effect of maternal alcohol consumption on CNS myelination in the developing rat.' Neuroscience Abstracts (Oxford), 11, 604.

770. HOLLOWAY, J.A. (1979) 'The fetal alcohol syndrome: Clinical and experimental studies.' Alcohol Technical Reports, 8, 9-12.

771. HOLLOWAY, J.A., and TAPP, W.N. (1978) 'Effects of prenatal and/or early postnatal exposure to ethanol on offspring of rats.' Alcohol Technical Reports, 7, 108-115.

772. HOLLSTEDT, C. (1975) 'Ger alkohol forsterskador?' ['Does alcohol injure the fetus?'] Alkohol och Narkotika, 69, 123-127.

773. HOLLSTEDT, C. (1981) 'Alcohol and the developing organism: Experimental and clinical studies.' Opuscula Medica, Supplementum 52, 1-24.

774. HOLLSTEDT, C., NERI, A., and RYDBERG, U. (1981) 'Ethanol-induced lethality in the developing rat.' Blutalkohol (in press).

775. HOLLSTEDT, C., OLSSON, O., and RYDBERG, U. (1977) 'The effect
      of alcohol on the developing organism: Genetical, terato-
      logical and physiological Aspects.' Medical Biology (Hel-
      sinki), 55, 1-14.

776. HOLLSTEDT, C., OLSSON, O., and RYDBERG, U. (1980) 'Effects of
      ethanol on the developing rat. II. Coordination as measured
      by the tilting-plane test.' Medical Biology (Helsinki), 58,
      164-168.

777. HOLLSTEDT, C., and RYDBERG, U. (1977) 'Alcohol and the de-
      veloping organism: Experimental and clinical aspects.'
      Excerpta Medica: International Congress Series, 407, 93-100.

778. HOLLSTEDT, C., RYDBERG, U., OLSSON, O., and BUIJTEN, J. (1980)
      'Effects of ethanol on the developing rat. I. Ethanol metab-
      olism and effects on lactate, pyruvate, and glucose concentra-
      tions.' Medical Biology (Helsinki), 58, 158-163.

779. HOOD, R.D., LARY, J.M., and BLACKLOCK, J.B. (1979) 'Lack of pre-
      natal effects of maternal ethanol consumption in CD-mice.'
      Toxicology Letters (Amsterdam), 4, 79-82.

780. HOOK, E.B. (1978) 'Dietary cravings and aversions during preg-
      nancy.' American Journal of Clinical Nutrition, 31, 1355-
      1362.

781. HOPPE, H. (1910) 'Procreation during intoxication.' (Translated
      and abridged by K.O. Brown.) Journal of Inebriety, 32, 105-
      110.

782. HOPPE, H. (1913) Die Tatsachen über den Alkohol. [The Facts con-
      cerning Alcohol.] 4th ed. Munich.

783. HORIGUCHI, T., SUZUKI, K., COMAS-URRUTIA, A.C., MUELLER-HEUBACH,
      E., BOYER-MILIC, A.M., BARATZ, R.A., MORISHIMA, H.O., JAMES,
      L.S., and ADAMSONS, K. (1971) 'Effect of ethanol upon
      uterine activity and fetal acid-base state in the rhesus
      monkey.' American Journal of Obstetrics and Gynecology, 109,
      910-917.

784. HORNSTEIN, L., CROWE, C., and GRUPPO, R. (1977) 'Adrenal car-
      cinoma in child with history of fetal alcohol syndrome.'
      Lancet (London), 2, 1292-1293.

785. HOROWITZ, J.D., and GOBLE, A.J. (1979) 'Drugs and impaired male
      sexual function.' Drugs, 18, 206-217.

786. HORROBIN, D.F. (1980) 'A biochemical basis for alcoholism and
      alcohol-induced damage including the fetal alcohol syndrome
      and cirrhosis: Interference with essential fatty acid and
      prostaglandin metabolism.' Medical Hypotheses, 6, 929-942.

787. HORTON, A.A.   (1978)   'Development of alcohol and aldehyde dehy-
      drogenase activities in rat liver.' British Journal of Alco-
      hol and Alcoholism, 13, 154-155.

788. HOSKINS, E.J., GULIZIA, G.W., and HOLLY, E.K.   (1981) 'Maternal
      ethanol and development of sympathetic tone in the newborn
      rat heart.' Research Communications in Substance Abuse, 2,
      127-134.

789. HOWE, S.G.   (1848)   Report Made to the Legislature of Massachusetts
      upon Idiocy. Boston: Coolidge and Wiley.

790. HOWE, S.G.   (1858)   On the Causes of Idiocy. Edinburgh and Lon-
      don.

791. HSIEH, D.P.H., SALHAB, A.S., WONG, J.J., and YANG, S.L.   (1974)
      'Toxicity of aflatoxin Q_1 as evaluated with the chicken em-
      bryo and bacterial auxotrophs.' Toxicology and Applied
      Pharmacology, 30, 237-242.

792. HUGOT, D., and CAUSERET, J.   (1978)   'Incidences de l'ingestion
      d'acide tannique, de métabisulfite de potassium et d'ethanol,
      administrés isolément ou en association, sur la reproduction
      chez la ratte.' ['Effects of ingestion of tannic acid, potas-
      sium metabisulfite and ethanol, administered alone or in com-
      bination, on the reproduction of the rat.'] Comptes Rendus
      des Seances de la Société de Biologie et des Filiales (Paris),
      172, 470-475.

793. HUGUES, J.N., PERRET, G., ADESSI, G., COSTE, T., and MODIGLIANI,
      E.   (1978)   'Effects of chronic alcoholism on the pituitary-
      gonadal function of women during menopausal transition and
      in the post menopausal period.' Biomedicine Express (Paris),
      29, 279-283.

794. HUME, A.R., DOUGLAS, B.H., and WHITE, E.L.   (1976)   'Placental
      transfer of ethyl alcohol.' International Research Commun-
      ications System (IRES) Medical Science: Library Compendium,
      4, 203.

795. HURLEY, L.S.   (1979)   'The fetal alcohol syndrome: Possible im-
      plications of nutrient deficiencies [and discussion].' In:
      Alcohol and Nutrition, Proceedings of a Workshop, Septem-
      ber 26-27, 1977, Indianapolis, Indiana (NIAAA Research
      Monograph No. 2). Ed. T.-K. Li, S. Schenker, and L. Lumeng.
      Washington, D.C.: U.S. Government Printing Office.

796. HÜTER, J., and SCHMITT, H.   (1968)   'Wehenhemmung mit Äthanol im
      Tierversuch.' ['Labor inhibition with ethanol in an animal
      experiment.'] Geburtshilfe und Frauenheilkunde (Stuttgart),
      28, 1050-1052.

797. HUTTUNEN, M.O., HÄRKÖNEN, M., NISKANEN, P., LEINO, T., and
      YLIKAHRI, R.   (1976)   'Plasma testosterone concentrations in
      alcoholics.' Journal of Studies on Alcohol, 37, 1165-1177.

I

798. IBER, F.L. (1980) 'Fetal alcohol syndrome.' Nutrition Today, 15, 4-11.

799. IDÄNPÄÄN-HEIKKILÄ, J.E., FRITCHIE, G.E., HO, B.T., and MC ISAAC, W.M. (1971) 'Placental transfer of C^{14}-ethanol.' American Journal of Obstetrics and Gynecology, 110, 426-428.

800. IDÄNPÄÄN-HEIKKILÄ, J.E., ISOAHO, R., and JOUPPILA, P. (1971) 'Placental transfer of ethanol and ethanol elimination rate in newborn and mother.' Scandinavian Journal of Clinical and Laboratory Investigation (Oslo), 27, 54.

801. IDÄNPÄÄN-HEIKKILÄ, J.E., JOUPPILA, P., AKERBLOM, H.K., ISOAHO, R., KAUPPILA, E., and KOIVISTO, M. (1972) 'Elimination and metabolic effects of ethanol in mother, fetus, and newborn infant.' American Journal of Obstetrics and Gynecology, 112, 387-393.

802. IGALI, S., and GAZSO, L. (1980) 'Mutagenic effect of alcohol and acetaldehyde on Escherichia coli.' Mutation Research (Amsterdam), 74, 209-210 (abstract).

803. IJAIYA, K., SCHWENK, A., and GLADTKE, E. (1976) 'Fetales Alkoholsyndrom.' ['Fetal alcohol syndrome.'] Deutsche Medizinische Wochenschrift (Stuttgart), 101, 1563-1568.

804. IJAIYA, K., SCHWENK, A., and GLADTKE, E. (1977) 'Missbildungen bei Kindern von Alkoholikerinnen.' [Malformations in children of women alcoholics.'] Schwestern Revue, 15, 20-23.

805. ILBERG, G. (1904) 'Sociale Psychiatrie.' ['Social psychiatry.'] Monatschrift für Soziale Medizin, 1, 321.

806. IL-INSKIKH, N.N., IL-INSKIKH, I.N., MAKAROV, L.N., and CHERNOSKUTOVA, S.A. (1978) 'Vlianiia etanola i yego metabolita atsetoal'degida na khromosomnii apparat kletok krysy i cheloveka.' ['Effect of ethanol and its metabolite acetaldehyde on the chromosomal apparatus of rat and human cells.'] Tsitologiia (Moscow), 20, 421-425.

807.   INOUE, K., and MASUDA, F. (1976) 'Effects of detergents on mouse
          fetuses.' Shokuhin Eiseigaku Zasshi [Journal of Food Hygiene
          Society of Japan], 17, 158-169.

808.   IOSUB, S., BINGOL, N., and FUCHS, M. (1975) 'Maternal alcoholism
          and fetal abnormalities.' Pedriatric Research, 9, 284 (ab-
          stract).

809.   IOSUB, S., FUCHS, M., BINGOL, N., and GROMISCH, D.S. (1980)
          'Fetal alcohol syndrome revisited.' Alcoholism: Clinical
          and Experimental Research, 4, 218 (abstract).

810.   IOSUB, S., FUCHS, M., BINGOL, N., and GROMISCH, D.S. (1981)
          'Fetal alcohol syndrome revisited.' Pediatrics, 68, 475-479.

811.   IOSUB, S., FUCHS, M., BINGOL, N., and STONE, R.K. (1981) 'Ef-
          fects of alcohol and narcotic abuse on the fetal heart.'
          Alcoholism: Clinical and Experimental Research, 5, 155 (ab-
          stract).

812.   IOSUB, S., FUCHS, M., BINGOL, N., STONE, R.K., and GROMISCH, D.S.
          (1981) 'Long-term follow-up of three siblings with fetal
          alcohol syndrome.' Alcoholism: Clinical and Experimental
          Research, 5, 523-527.

813.   IOSUB, S., FUCHS, M., BINGOL, N., and WASSERMAN, E. (1981) 'Ef-
          fects of ethanol and opiates on sex ratio in FAS.' Alco-
          holism: Clinical and Experimental Research, 5, 154 (ab-
          stract).

814.   IVANOV, J. (1912) 'Der Einfluss des Alkohols auf die Spermatozen
          von Säugetieren und Befruchtungsversuche mit Sperma unter Zu-
          satz von Alkohol.' ['The influence of alcohol on the sper-
          matozoa of mammals and attempts at fertilization with sperms
          under the condition of alcohol.'] Münchener Medizinische
          Wochenschrift (Munich), 18, 998.

815.   IVANOV, J. (1913) 'Action de l'alcool sur les spermatozoïdes
          des mammifères.' ['Action of alcohol on the spermatozoa of
          mammals.'] Comptes Rendus des Seances de la Société de Bio-
          logie et de ses Filiales (Paris), 74, 480-482.

816.   IVANOV, J. (1913) 'Expériences sur la fécondation des mammi-
          fères avec le sperme mélange d'alcool.' ['Experiences on
          the impregnation of mammals with sperm mixed with alcohol.']
          Comptes Rendus des Seances de la Société de Biologie et de
          ses Filiales (Paris), 74, 482-484.

817.   IWASE, N.T., TAKAHASHI, M., and KOMURA, S. (1979) 'An exper-
          imental study of the fetal alcohol syndrome in neonatal
          mouse brain.' Arukoru Kenkyu, 14, 286.

818.   IWASE, N.T., TSUJI, M., TAKAHASHI, S., and KOMURA, S.   (1980)
       'An experimental study of the fetal alcohol syndrome using
       an animal model with mice: Neurochemical determination of
       monoamines, polyamines, and nucleic acids in neonatal
       brain.' [Japanese.] Nippon Arukoru Igakkai [Japanese
       Journal of Studies on Alcohol, 15, 9-18.

J

819. J., E. (1849) 'Reports on idiocy.' American Journal of the
      Medical Sciences, 17, 421-441.

820. JACOBSON, S., RICH, J'A., and TOVSKY, N.J. (1978) 'Retardation
      of cerebral cortical development as a consequence of the
      fetal alcohol syndrome.' Alcoholism: Clinical and Exper-
      imental Research, 2, 193.

821. JACOBSON, S., RICH, J'A., and TOVSKY, N.J. (1979) 'Delayed
      myelination and lamination in the cerebral cortex of the al-
      bino rat as a result of the fetal alcohol syndrome.' In:
      Currents in Alcoholism. Volume 5: Biomedical Issues and
      Clinical Effects of Alcoholism. Ed. M. Galanter. New York:
      Grune and Stratton, pp. 123-133.

822. JACOBSON, S., SEHGAL, P., BRONSON, R., DOOR, B., and BURNAP, J.
      (1980) 'Comparisons between an oral and an intravenous method
      to demonstrate the in utero effects of ethanol in the monkey.'
      Neurobehavioral Toxicology, 2, 253-258.

823. JACOBSON, S., SEHGAL, P., BRONSON, R., DOOR, B., KLEPPER-KILGORE,
      N., and BURNAP, J. (1980) 'A non-human primate model to
      demonstrate the teratogenic effects of ethanol.' Teratology,
      21, 45A-46A (abstract).

824. JACOBSON, S., SEHGAL, P.,,, BRONSON, R., MC CLURE, R., and KLEPPER-
      KILGORE, N. (1980) 'Behavioral abnormalities as a consequence
      of in utero exposure to ethanol in the monkey, macaca fascicu-
      laris.' Alcoholism: Clinical and Experimental Research, 4,
      219 (abstract).

825. JACOBSON, S., TROXELL, S., SEHGAL, P., BRONSON, R., BURNAP, J.,
      and KLEPPER-KILGORE, N. (1981) 'Developmental delay and
      behavioral abnormalities as a consequence of in utero ex-
      posure to ethanol in the monkey.' Alcoholism: Clinical and
      Experimental Research, 5, 155 (abstract).

826. JAKUBOVIC, A., MC GEER, P.L., and FITZSIMMONS, R.C. (1976) 'Effects of delta 9-tetrahydrocannabinol and ethanol on body weight protein and nucleic acid synthesis in chick embryos.' Journal of Toxicology and Environmental Health, 1, 441-447.

827. JEWETT, J.F. (1976) 'Committee on maternal welfare: Alcoholism and ruptured uterus.' New England Journal of Medicine, 294, 335-336.

828. JOFFE, J.M. (1979) 'Influence of drug exposure of the father on perinatal outcome.' Clinics in Perinatology, 6, 21-36.

829. JOHN, J.A.,SMITH, F.A., LEONG, B.K.J., and SCHWETZ, B.A. (1977) 'Effects of maternally inhaled vinyl chloride on embryonal and fetal development in mice, rats, and rabbits.' Toxicology and Applied Pharmacology, 39, 497-513.

830. JOHNSON, C.F. (1974) 'Does maternal alcoholism affect offspring?' Clinical Pedriatrics, 13, 633-634.

831. JOHNSON, K.G. (1979) 'Fetal alcohol syndrome: Rhinorrhea, persistent otitis media, choanal stenosis, hydroplastic sphenoids and ethmoid.' Rocky Mountain Medical Journal, 76, 64-65.

832. JOHNSON, S., and GARZON, S.R. (1978) 'Alcoholism and women.' American Journal of Drug and Alcohol Abuse, 5, 107-122.

833. JOHNSON, S., KNIGHT, R., MARMER, D.J., and STEELE, R.W. (1981) 'Immune deficiency in fetal alcohol syndrome.' Pediatric Research, 15, 908-911.

834. JONES, B.M., and JONES, M.K. (1976) 'Alcohol effects in women during the menstrual cycle.' Annals of the New York Academy of Sciences, 273, 576-587.

835. JONES, B.M., and JONES, M.K. (1976) 'Women and alcohol: Intoxication, metabolism, and the menstrual cycle.' In: Alcoholism Problems in Women and Children. Ed. M. Greenblatt and M.A. Schuckit. New York: Grune and Stratton, pp. 103-136.

836. JONES, B.M., JONES, M.K., and HATCHER, E.M. (1980) 'Cognitive deficits in women alcoholics as a function of gynecological status.' Journal of Studies on Alcohol, 41, 140-146.

837. JONES, C.T., BODDY, K., and ROBINSON, J.S. (1977) Changes in the concentration of adrenocorticotrophin and corticosteroid in the plasma of foetal sheep in the latter half of pregnancy and during labor.' Journal of Endocrinology (London), 72, 293-300.

838. JONES, K.L. (1975) 'Aberrant neuronal migration in the fetal alcohol syndrome.' Birth Defects, 11, 131-132.

839. JONES, K.L. (1975) 'The fetal alcohol syndrome.' Addictive
      Diseases, 2, 79-88.

840. JONES, K.L. (1977) 'Fetal alcohol syndrome.' In: Drug Abuse
      in Pregnancy and Neonatal Effects. Ed. J.L. Rementeria.
      St. Louis: C.V. Mosby Company, pp. 117-164.

841. JONES, K.L. (1980) 'State of the art address: Clinical
      studies--dysmorphology.' Paper presented at the Fetal Alco-
      hol Syndrome Workshop, Seattle, Washington (May 2-4).

842. JONES, K.L., and CHERNOFF, G.F. (1978) 'Drugs and chemicals as-
      sociated with intrauterine growth deficiency.' Journal of
      Reproductive Medicine, 21, 365-370.

843. JONES, K.L., HANSON, J.W., and SMITH, D.W. (1978) 'Palpebral
      fissure size in newborn infants.' Journal of Pedriatrics,
      92, 787.

844. JONES, K.L., and SMITH, D.W. (1973) 'Recognition of the fetal
      alcohol syndrome in early infancy.' Lancet (London), 2, 999-
      1001.

845. JONES, K.L., and SMITH, D.W. (1974) 'Offspring of chronic alco-
      holic women.' Lancet (London), 2, 349.

846. JONES, K.L., and SMITH, D.W. (1975) 'The fetal alcohol syn-
      drome.' Teratology, 12, 1-10.

847. JONES, K.L., and SMITH, D.W. (1978) 'Effects of alcohol on the
      fetus.' [Letter.] New England Journal of Medicine, 298,
      55-56.

848. JONES, K.L., SMITH, D.W., and HANSON, J.W. (1976) 'The fetal
      alcohol syndrome: Clinical delineation.' Annals of the
      New York Academy of Sciences, 273, 130-137.

849. JONES, K.L., SMITH, D.W., OUELLETTE, E.M., KAMINSKI, M., RUMEAU-
      ROUQUETTE, C., and SCHWARTZ, D. (1978) 'Effects of alcohol
      on the fetus.' New England Journal of Medicine, 298, 55-56.

850. JONES, K.L., SMITH, D.W., and STREISSGUTH, A. (1974) 'Incidence
      of the fetal alcohol syndrome in offspring of chronically
      alcoholic women.' Pediatric Research, 84, 440.

851. JONES, K.L., SMITH, D.W., STREISSGUTH, A.P., and MYRIANTHOPOULOS,
      N.C.(1974) 'Outcome in offspring of chronic alcoholic women.'
      Lancet (London), 1, 1076-1078.

852. JONES, K.L., SMITH, D.W., ULLELAND, C.N., and STREISSGUTH, A.P.
      (1973) 'Pattern of malformation in offspring of chronic
      alcoholic mothers.' Lancet (London), 1, 1267-1271.

853. JONES, M.K., TARTER, R.E., and JONES, B.M. (1981) 'The effects
      of the menstrual cycle on craving in female alcoholics.'
      Alcoholism: Clinical and Experimental Research, 5, 156
      (abstract).

854. JONES, P.J.H., LEICHTER, J., and LEE, M. (1981) 'Placental
      blood flow in rats fed alcohol before and during gestation.'
      Life Sciences, 29, 1153-1159.

855. JONES, P.J.H., LEICHTER, J., and LEE, M. (1981) 'Uptake of zinc,
      folate, and analogs of glucose and amino acid by the rat
      fetus exposed to alcohol in utero.' Nutrition Reports Inter-
      national, 24, 75-83.

856. JOUPPILA, P., HUIKKO, M., and JÄRVINEN, P.A. (1970) 'Effect of
      ethyl alcohol on urinary excretion of noradrenaline and
      adrenaline in patients with threatened premature delivery.'
      Acta Obstetrica et Gynecologica Scandinavica (Lund), 49,
      359-362.

857. JOYNT, R. (1974-1975) 'Mental retardation and alcoholism.'
      Pointer, 21, 76.

858. JÓŹWIK, T. (1972) 'Rozmieszczenie etanolu u płodu w przypadku
      ostrego zatrucia kobiety ciężarnej.' ['Distribution of alco-
      hol in foetus in a case of acute ethanol poisoning of the
      pregnant woman.'] Archiwum Medycyny Sądowej i Kryminologii,
      22, 243-245.

859. JUNG, A.L., ROAN, Y., and TEMPLE, A.R. (1980) 'Neonatal death
      associated with acute transplacental ethanol intoxication.'
      American Journal of Diseases in Children, 134, 419-420.

K

860. KABBHEL, G. (1909) 'Über den Einfluss des Alkohols auf das Keim-
      plasma.' ['Concerning the influence of alcohol on cell plas-
      ma.'] Archiv für Hygiene, 71, 124-130.

861. KAHN, A.J. (1968) 'Effect of ethanol exposure during embryo-
      genesis and the neonatal period on the incidence of hepatoma
      in C_3H male mice.' Growth, 32, 311-316.

862. KAHN, E. (1981) 'Attention deficit syndrome in children born to
      alcoholic mothers.' [Letter.] Journal of Pediatrics, 98,
      670-671.

863. KAKIHANA, R., AND BUTTE, J.C. (1980) 'Steroid hormone effects
      of ethyl alcohol consumption in pregnant rats and their off-
      spring.' Paper presented at the 20th Annual Meeting of the
      Teratology Society, Portsmouth, New Hampshire (June 8-12).

864. KAKIHANA, R., BUTTE, J.C., and MOORE, J.P. (1979) 'Neuroendo-
      crine effects of maternal alcoholization: Plasma and cor-
      terosterone in neonatal rats.' Alcoholism: Clinical and
      Experimental Research, 3, 182 (abstract).

865. KAKIHANA, R., BUTTE, J.C., and MOORE, J.A. (1980) 'Endocrine
      effects of maternal alcoholization: Plasma and brain testos-
      terone dihydrotestosterone, estradiol and corticostone.'
      Alcoholism: Clinical and Experimental Research, 4, 57-61.

866. KALIN, R., MC CLELLAND, D.C., and KAHN, M. (1972) 'The effects
      of male social drinking in fantasy.' In: The Drinking Man.
      Ed. D.C. Mc Clelland, W.N. Davis, R. Kalin, and E. Wanner.
      New York: The Free Press, pp. 3-20.

867. KAMATH, S.H., and WAZIRI, R. (1978) 'The progeny of alcoholic
      rats.' Alcoholism: Clinical and Experimental Research, 2,
      216 (abstract).

868. KAMINSKI, M. (1980) 'Three French surveys on the effects of mod-
      erate alcohol use in pregnancy.' Paper presented at the Fe-
      tal Alcohol Syndrome Workshop, Seattle, Washington (May 2-4).

869. KAMINSKI, M., FRANC, M., LEBOUVIER, M., DU MAZAUBRUN, C., and
      RUMEAU-ROUQUETTE, C. (1981) 'Moderate alcohol use and preg-
      nancy outcome.' Neurobehavioral Toxicology and Teratology, 3,
      173-181.

870. KAMINSKI, M., GOUJARD, J., RUMEAU-ROUQUETTE, C., and SCHWARTZ, D.
      (1978) 'Maternal smoking, alcohol consumption, and abruptio
      placentae.' [Letter.] American Journal of Obstetrics and
      Gynecology, 130, 738-739.

871. KAMINSKI, M., RUMEAU-ROUQUETTE, C., and SCHWARTZ, D. (1975) 'La
      consommation d'alcool chez les femmes enceintes et son effets
      sur l'issue de la grossesse.' ['Alcohol consumption in preg-
      nant women and its effects on the outcome of pregnancy.']
      INSERM/MRC, 54, 87-100.

872. KAMINSKI, M., RUMEAU-ROUQUETTE, C., and SCHWARTZ, D. (1976) 'Con-
      summation d'alcool chez les femmes enceintes et issue de la
      grossesse.' Revue d'Epidemiologie, Médecine Sociale et de
      Santé Publique (Paris), 24, 27-40. (Translated into English
      in 1978 by R.E. Little and A. Schinzel: 'Alcohol consumption
      in pregnant women and the outcome of pregnancy.' Alcoholism:
      Clinical and Experimental Research, 2, 155-163.)

873. KAMINSKI, M., RUMEAU-ROUQUETTE, C., and SCHWARTZ, D. (1977) 'Con-
      sommation d'alcool chez les femmes enceintes et etat de l'en-
      fant à la naissance.' ['Consumption of alcohol by pregnant
      women and the condition of the infant at birth.'] Notes
      d'Études Documentation, No. 4396-4397-4398, pp. 73-75.

874. KAMINSKI, M., RUMEAU-ROUQUETTE, C., and SCHWARTZ, D. (1978) 'Ef-
      fects of alcohol on the fetus.' [Letter.] New England Jour-
      nal of Medicine, 298, 55-56.

875. KAMINSKI, M., RUMEAU-ROUQUETTE, C., and SCHWARTZ, D. (1979) 'Re-
      sponse to questions re: "Alcohol consumption in pregnant
      women and the outcome of pregnancy,"' translated by R.E. Lit-
      tle and S. Quinn. Alcoholism: Clinical and Experimental Re-
      search, 3, 92.

876. KARACAN, I., SNYDER, S., SALIS, P.J., WILLIAMS, R.L., and DER-
      MAN, S. (1980) 'Sexual dysfunction in male alcoholics and
      its objective evaluation.' In: Phenomenology and Treatment
      of Alcoholism. Ed. W.E. Fann, I. Karacan, A.D. Pokorny, and
      R.L. Williams. New York: SP Medical and Scientific Books,
      pp. 259-268.

877. KARU, E.Y. (1980) 'Po povodu stat: F.I. Stekhuna "Vliyaniye
      alkogolya na muzhskiye polovyye zhelezy."' ['Comment on
      F.I. Stekhun's paper: "Effects of alcohol on male sexual
      glands."'] Zhurnal Nevropatologie, 80, 131-132.

878. KAWAJI, K., OTA, S., and BABA, T.   (1940)   'Experimentelle Erzeu-
          gung der Missbildung.'   ['Experimental generation of malfor-
          mation.']   Nippon Byori Gakkai Zasshi [Transactions of the
          Society of Pathology in Japan], 30, 499.

879. KAYUSHEVA, I.V.   (1979)   'Alkogolizam i endokrinnaye sistema.'
          ['Alcohol and the endocrine system.']   Sovetskaya Meditsina
          (Moscow), 72, 87-91.

880. KENNEDY, L.A.   (1977)   'Teratological evaluation of ethanol,
          pentobarbital, and combinations of these in the rat.'
          Ph.D. Thesis, University of Manitoba, Canada.

881. KENNEDY, L.A.   (1981)   'The health and fecundity of mice fed a
          "nutritionally adequate" liquid diet.'   Anatomical Record,
          199, 148 (abstract).

882. KENNEDY, L.A., and PERSAUD, T.V.N.   (1978)   'Prenatal toxicity of
          simultaneously administered ethanol and pentobarbital in the
          rat.'   Experimental Pathology (Jena), 15, 250-259.

883. KENNEDY, L.A., and PERSAUD, T.V.N.   (1979)   'Acute alcohol intox-
          ication in the pregnant rat.'   In: Teratological Testing.
          Ed. T.V.N. Persaud. Baltimore, Maryland: University Park
          Place, pp. 223-238 [also in Advanced Study in Birth Defects,
          2, 223-238].

884. KENT, J.R., SCARAMUZZI, R.J., and LAUWERS, W.   (1973)   'Plasma
          testosterone, estradiol and gonadotropins in hepatic insuf-
          ficiency.'   Gastroenterology, 64, 111-115.

885. KENT, W.C., and WHITNEY, J.E.   (1981)   'Effect of ethanol or acet-
          aldehyde on lipid biosynthesis in human umbilical artery.'
          Federation Proceedings, 40, 803 (abstract).

886. KESÄNIEMI, A.   (1974)   'Studies in the ethanol-combined galactose
          elimination test with special reference to pregnancy.'   Dis-
          sertation, University of Helsinki.

887. KESÄNIEMI, Y.A.   (1974)   'Ethanol and acetaldehyde in the milk and
          peripheral blood of lactating women after ethanol adminis-
          tration.'   Journal of Obstetrics and Gynaecology of the Brit-
          ish Commonwealth, 81, 84-86.

888. KESÄNIEMI, Y.A.   (1974)   'Metabolism of ethanol and acetaldehyde
          in intact rats during pregnancy.'   Biochemical Pharmacology,
          23, 1157-1162.

889. KESÄNIEMI, Y.A., KURPPA, K.O., and HUSMAN, K.R.H.   (1973)   'Eth-
          anol-combined galactose tolerance test in healthy pregnant
          women and the effect of a high-protein diet.'   Journal of Ob-
          stetrics and Gynaecology of the British Commonwealth, 80,
          344-348.

890. KESÄNIEMI, Y.A., KURPPA, K.O., and SALASPURO, M.P. (1973) 'Comparison of intravenous and peroral galactose elimination test with and without ethanol in different clinical conditions.' Scandinavian Journal of Gastroenterology (Oslo), 8, 593-598.

891. KESÄNIEMI, Y.A., and SIPPEL, H.W. (1975) 'Placental and foetal metabolism of acetaldehyde in rat. I. Contents of ethanol and acetaldehyde in placenta and foetus of the pregnant rat during ethanol oxidation.' Acta Pharmacologica et Toxicologica (Copenhagen), 37, 43-48.

892. KESSEL, N. (1977) 'The fetal alcohol syndrome from the public health study point.' Health Trends, 9, 86.

893. KEYNES, J.M. (1910-1911) 'Influence of parental alcoholism.' Journal of the Royal Statistical Society, 74, 339-345.

894. KHAMOV, S.V. (1976) 'Vliianie alkogolia na potomstvo.' ['Effects of alcohol on progeny.] Fel'dsher i Akusherka, 41, 33-36.

895. KHAN, A., BADER, J.L., HOY, G.R., and SINKS, L.F. (1979) 'Hepatoblastoma in child with fetal alcohol syndrome.' [Letter.] Lancet (London), 1, 1403-1404.

896. KHAWAJA, J.A., WALLGREN, H., OSMI, H., and HILSKA, P. (1978) 'Neuronal and liver protein synthesis in the developing offspring following treatment of pregnant rats with ethanol or 1,3-butanediol.' Research Communications in Chemical Pathology and Pharmacology, 22, 573-580.

897. KHVATOV, B.P. (1975) 'Eksperimentalnie dannie o bliyanii alkogolya na oplodotvorenie.' ['Experimental data on the effect of alcohol in fertilization.'] Byulleten Eksperimentalnoi Biologii i Meditsiny, 79, 106-107.

898. KIEBOOMS, L. (1979) 'Abortus en het foetale alcohol syndroom.' ['Abortion and the fetal alcohol syndrome' (Letter).] South African Medical Journal (Cape Town), 55, 155.

899. KIEFFER, J.D., and KETCHEL, M.M. (1970) 'Blockade of ovulation in the rat by ethanol.' Acta Endocrinologica (Copenhagen), 65, 117-124.

900. KIM, S.S., and HODGKINSON, R. (1976) 'Acute ethanol intoxication and its prolonged effect on a full-term neonate.' Anesthesia and Analgesia: Current Researches, 55, 602-603.

901. KINNEY, H., FAIX, R., and BRAZY, J. (1980) 'The fetal alcohol syndrome and neuroblastoma.' Pediatrics, 66, 130-132.

902. KINSEY, B.A. (1966) The Female Alcoholic: A Social Psychological Study. Springfield, Illinois: Charles C. Thomas.

903. KINSEY, B.A. (1968) 'Psychological factors in alcoholic women
         from a state hospital sample.' American Journal of Psychi-
         atry, 124, 1463-1466.

904. KIRCHNER, M. (1979) 'Das embryonale Alkoholsyndrom.' ['Embryo-
         nal alcohol syndrome.'] Kinderärtzliche Praxis, 47, 574-
         584.

905. KIRKPATRICK, S.E., PITLICK, P.T., HIRSCHKLAU, M.J., and FRIED-
         MAN, W.F. (1976) 'Acute effects of maternal ethanol in-
         fusion on fetal cardiac performance.' American Journal of
         Obstetrics and Gynecology, 126, 1034-1037.

906. KLASSEN, R.W., and PERSAUD, T.V.N. (1976) 'Experimental studies
         on the influence of male alcoholism on pregnancy and pro-
         geny.' Experimentelle Pathologie (Jena), 12, 38-45.

907. KLASSEN, R.W., and PERSAUD, T.V.N. (1978) 'Influence of alcohol
         on the reproductive system of the male rat.' International
         Journal of Fertility, 23, 176-184.

908. KLASSEN, R.W., and PERSAUD, T.V.N. (1979) 'Experimental studies
         on the influence of male alcoholism on testicular function,
         pregnancy, and progeny.' Advanced Study in Birth Defects, 2,
         239-256.

909. KLEY, H.K., STROHMEYER, G., and KRUSKEMPER, H.L. (1979) 'Effect
         of testosterone application on hormone concentrations of andro-
         gens and estrogens in male patients with cirrhosis of the
         liver.' Gastroenterology, 76, 235-241.

910. KLINE, J. (1980) 'Moderate alcohol use and spontaneous abortions:
         A case-control study.' Paper presented at the Fetal Alcohol
         Syndrome Workshop, Seattle, Washington (May 2-4).

911. KLINE, J., SHROUT, P., STEIN, Z., SUSSER, M., and WARBURTON, D.
         (1980) 'Drinking during pregnancy and spontaneous abortion.'
         Lancet (London), 2, 176-180.

912. KNÖRR, K. (1979) 'Der Einfluss von Tabak und Alkohol auf Schwang-
         erschaftsverlauf und Kindesentwicklung.' ['The effect of
         tobacco and alcohol on the course of pregnancy and on child
         development.'] Bulletin der Schweizerischen Akademie der Med-
         izinischen Wissenschaften, 35, 137-146.

913. KODA, L.Y., SHOEMAKER, W.J., and BLOOM, F.E. (1980) 'Toxic ef-
         fects of alcohol on the chicken embryo.' Alcoholism: Clin-
         ical and Experimental Research, 4, 220 (abstract).

914. KODA, L.Y., SHOEMAKER, W.J., SHOEMAKER, C.A., and BLOOM, F.E.
         (1980) 'Toxic effects of ethanol on the chicken embryo.'
         Substance and Alcohol Actions/Misuse, 1, 343-350.

915. KOLATA, G.B. (1978) 'Teratogens acting through males.' Sci-
         ence, 202, 733 (abstract).

916.   KOLATA, G.B.   (1981)   'Fetal alcohol advisory debated.'   Science, 214, 642-643, 645.

917.   KOLLER, B.   (1891)   Über die Einwirkung von Geburt an Gerichter steigender Alkoholgaben auf den Organismus junger Hunde. [On the Effect from Birth of Adjusted Increasing Alcohol Doses on the System of Young Dogs.]   Basel.

918.   KOLLER, J.   (1895)   'Beitrag zur Erblichkeitsstatistik der Geisteskranken im Kanton Zurich.'   ['Report on nausea statistics of the mentally ill in the canton of Zurich.']   Archiv für Psychiatrie (Berlin), 27, 268-294.

919.   KOMURA, S., NIIMI, Y., and YOSHITAKE, Y.   (1970)   'Alcohol preference during reproductive cycle in female C57Bl mice. 1. Relationship between alcohol preference and liver alcohol dehydrogenase activity.'   Japanese Journal of Studies on Alcohol, 5, 91-96.

920.   KORÁNYI, G.   (1977)   'Embryopathia alcoholica.'   ['Alcoholic embryopathy.']   Orvosi Hetilap (Budapest), 118, 504-507.

921.   KORÁNYI, G.   (1978)   'Embryopathia alcoholica.'   ['Embryopathia alcoholica.']   Alkohologia (Budapest), 9, 70-75.

922.   KORÁNYI, G., and OSIKY, E.   (1978)   'Az embryopathia alcoholica gyermekkorban észlelheto tüneteiről.'   ['Symptoms of alcoholic embryopathy noticeable in childhood.']   Orvosi Hetilap (Budapest), 119, 2923-2929.

923.   KORÁNYI, G., and OSIKY, E.   (1978)   'Signs of alcoholic embryopathy diagnosed in childhood.'   Orvosi Hetilap (Budapest), 119, 2923-2929.

924.   KORNGUTH, S.E., RUTLEDGE, J.J., SUNDERLAND, E., SIEGEL, F., CARLSON, I., SMOLLENS, J., JUHL, U., and YOUNG, B.   (1979)   'Impeded cerebellar development and reduced serum thyroxine levels associated with fetal alcohol intoxication.'   Brain Research, 177, 347-360.

925.   KORTE, A., SLACIK-ERBEN, R., and OBE, G.   (1979)   'The influence of ethanol treatment on cytogenetic effects in bone marrow cells of Chinese hamsters by cyclophosphamide, aflatoxin B_1 and patulin.'   Toxicology (Amsterdam), 12, 53-61.

926.   KOSTITCH, A.   (1922)   'Action de l'alcool sur les cellules seminales.'   ['Alcohol action on seminal cells.']   Revue Internationale contra l'Alcoolesmi, 30, 53-70.

927.   KOTZIN, M.   (1977)   'Fetal alcohol syndrome.'   Media and Methods, 14, 23.

928.   KOURI, M., KOIVULA, T., and KOIVUSALO, M.   (1977)   'Aldehyde dehydrogenase activity in human placenta.'   Acta Pharmacologica et Toxicologica (Copenhagen), 40, 460-464.

929. KOVACH, J.K. (1967) 'Maternal behavior in the domestic cock
      under the influence of alcohol.' Science, 156, 835-837.

930. KRASNER, J., ERIKKSSON, M., and YAFFE, S.J. (1974) 'Developmen-
      tal changes in mouse liver alcohol dehydrogenase.' Bio-
      chemical Pharmacology, 23, 519-522.

931. KRONICK, J.B. (1976) 'Teratogenic effects of ethyl alcohol admin-
      istered to pregnant mice.' American Journal of Obstetrics and
      Gynecology, 124, 676-680.

932. KRŠIAK, M., ELLIS, J., PÖSCHLOVÁ, N., and MASEK, K. (1977) 'In-
      creased aggressiveness and lower brain serotonin levels in
      offspring of mice given alcohol during gestation.' Journal
      of Studies on Alcohol, 38, 1696-1704.

933. KULLER, L.H., MAY, S.J., and PERPER, J.A. (1978) 'The relation-
      ship between alcohol, liver disease, and testicular path-
      ology.' American Journal of Epidemiology, 108, 192-199.

934. KUMAR, R., and BIJLANI, V. (1980) 'Foetal alcohol syndrome.'
      Indian Pediatrics, 17, 195-197.

935. KUMAR, S., and RAWAT, A.K. (1977) 'Prolonged ethanol consumption
      by pregnant and lactating rats and its effect on cerebral
      dopamine in the fetus and the neonate.' Research Communica-
      tions in Psychology, Psychiatry and Behavior, 2, 259-278.

936. KUNIKOVSKAYA, L.S. (1975) 'Effect of chronic alcoholic intox-
      ication on the respiratory enzymes in the tissues of newborn
      offspring.' [In Russian.] Zdravookjranenie, 18, 11-13.

937. KUNIKOVSKAYA, L.S. (1980) 'Klinicheskaya kharakteristika oligo-
      frenii alkogol'no-émbriopaticheskogo geneza.' ['Clinical
      characteristics of mental retardation of alcoholic-embryopathic
      origin.'] Zhurnal Nevropatologii i Psikhiatrii, 80, 417-422.

938. KUSS, J.-J., FISCHBACH, M., STOLL, C., and LÉVY, J.-M. (1979)
      'Effets conjugués sur le foetus de l'éthanol et des anti-
      épileptiques; à propos de 2 observations.' ['Combined effects
      of ethanol and antiepileptics on the fetus: Apropos of 2
      cases.' Pédiatrie, 34, 333-339.

939. KUZMA, J.W. (1980) 'The Loma Linda study.' Paper presented at
      the Fetal Alcohol Syndrome Workshop, Seattle, Washington
      (May 2-4).

940. KUZMA, J.W., and KISSINGER, D.G. (1981) 'Patterns of alcohol
      and cigarette use in pregnancy.' Neurobehavioral Toxicology
      and Teratology, 3, 211-221.

941. KUZMA, J.W., and PHILLIPS, R.L. (1976) 'Characteristics of
      drinking and non-drinking mothers.' Presented at the 104th
      Annual Meeting of the American Public Health Association,
      Miami, Florida.

942.   KUZMA, J.W., and PHILLIPS, R.L.   (1977)   'Characteristics of
         drinking and non-drinking mothers and their offspring.'
         Alcoholism: Clinical and Experimental Research, 1, 163.

943.   KYLLERMAN, M., OLEGÅRD, R., and SABEL, K.G.   (1977)   'Fetal alco-
         hol syndrome.' [Letter to the editor.] Developmental Med-
         icine and Child Neurology (London), 19, 695.

944.   KYRLE, J., and SCHOPPER, K.J.   (1914)   'Untersuchungen über den
         Einfluss des Alkohols auf Liber und Hoden des Kaminchen.'
         ['Studies concerning the influence of alcohol on the liver and
         testicle of the rabbit.'] Virchows Archiv, 215, 309-335.

L

946.   LAALE, H. W. (1971) 'Ethanol induced notochord and spinal
        cord duplications in the embryo of the zebra fish,
        "Brachydanio rerio." Journal of Experimental Zoology,
        177, 51-64.

947.   LAGERSPETZ, K. (1972). 'Postnatal development of the effects
        of alcohol and of the induced tolerance to alcohol in
        mice.' Pharmacologica et Toxicologica, 31, 497-508.

948.   LAITINEN, T. (1907) 'Uber die Einwirkung der kleinsten
        Alkoholmengen auf die Widerstandsfahigkeit des tier-
        ischen Organismus mit besonderer Berucksichtigung
        der Nachkommenschaft.' (On the effect of the
        smallest amount of alcohol on the robustness of the
        animal organism with special attention to the offspring.')
        Zeitschrift fur Hygiene und Infektionskrankheiten,
        58, 139-164.

949.   LAITENEN, T. (9109) 'A contribution to the study of
        the influence of alcohol on the degeneration of human
        offspring.' Proceedings of the Twelfth International
        Congress on Alcoholism (London), 263-270.

950.   LAMACHE, A. (1967) 'Reflexions sur la descendance des
        alcoolismes.' ('Reflections on the offspring of alcoholics.')
        (Letter). Bulletin de l'Academie Nationale de Medecine,
        151, 517-521.

951.   LAMBERT, G. H., PAPP, L. A., and NISHIURA, B. (1979) 'Disulfiram
        (D) and the fetal alcohol syndrome (FAS).' Pediatric
        Research, 14, 586 (abstract #961).

952. LANDESMAN-DWYER, S. (1980) 'Moderate drinking and 4-year-old
          development.' Paper presented at the Fetal Alcohol Syndrome
          Workshop, Seattle, Washington (May 2-4).

953. LANDESMAN-DWYER, S. (1981) 'The relationship of children's be-
          havior to maternal alcohol consumption.' In: Fetal Alcohol
          Syndrome, Volume 2: Human Studies. Ed. E.L. Abel. Boca
          Raton, Florida: CRC Press (in press).

954. LANDESMAN-DWYER, S., and KELLER, L.S. (1977) 'Naturalistic ob-
          servation of high and low risk newborns.' Alcoholism: Clin-
          ical and Experimental Research, 2, 177-178 (abstract).

955. LANDESMAN-DWYER, S., KELLER, L.S., and STREISSGUTH, A.P. (1978)
          'Naturalistic observations of newborns: Effects of maternal
          alcohol intake.' Alcoholism: Clinical and Experimental
          Research, 2, 171-177.

956. LANDESMAN-DWYER, S., KELLER, L., and STREISSGUTH, A.P. (1978)
          'Naturalistic observations of newborns: Effects of maternal
          alcohol intake. Reply to Drs. Sanders, Haynes, and Emde's
          review.' Sleep Reviews, 169, 36-39.

957. LANDESMAN-DWYER, S., RAGOZIN, A.S., and LITTLE, R.E. (1980)
          'Behavioral correlates of prenatal exposure to ethanol.'
          Teratology, 21, 52A (abstract).

958. LANDESMAN-DWYER, S., RAGOZIN, A.S., and LITTLE, R.E. (1981) 'Be-
          havioral correlates of prenatal alcohol exposure: A four-
          year follow-up study.' Neurobehavioral Toxicology and Tera-
          tology, 3, 187-193.

959. LANDESMAN-DWYER, S., and SCHUCKIT, M.A. (1978) 'Alcoholism and
          Down's syndrome.' Alcoholism: Clinical and Experimental
          Research, 2, 216 (abstract).

960. LANDESMAN-DWYER, S., SULZBACHER, F.M., and SCHUCKIT, M.A. (1978)
          'Down's Syndrome, maternal alcoholism, and accelerated bio-
          logic aging.' Alcoholism and Drug Abuse Institute Technical
          Report, University of Washington, Seattle, Washington, #78-19.

961. LANDOWSKI, J., and GILL, J. (1964) 'Einige Beobachtungen über
          das Sperma des Indischen Elefanten (Elephas maximum L.).'
          ['A few observations on the sperm of Indian elephants
          (Elephas maximum L.).'] Zoologische Garten (Leipzig),
          29, 205.

962. LANG, A.R. (1978) 'Sexual guilt, expectancies and alcohol as
          determinants of interest in and reaction to sexual stimuli.'
          Ph.D. Dissertation, University of Wisconsin-Madison.

963. LANNING, J.C. (1980) 'Effects of ethanol on human fetal cerebral
          cortex in vitro.' Anatomical Record, 196, 242.

964. LANNING, J.C. (1981) 'The effects of ethanol on human fetal
      cerebral cortex in vitro.' Dissertation Abstracts Inter-
      national, 41, 2436-B (abstract).

965. LARSSON, G. (1979) 'Försöksverksamhet i Stockholm: Att inom
      mödravarden ta hand om gravida missbrukare.' ['Abuse of alco-
      hol and drugs at maternal health clinics.'] Alkohol och Nar-
      kotika, 73, 19-25.

966. LAU, C., THADANI, P.V., SCHANBERG, S.M., and SLOTKIN, T.A. (1976)
      'Effects of maternal ethanol ingestion on development of
      adrenal catecholamines and dopamine-β-hydroxylase in the off-
      spring.' Neuropharmacology (Oxford), 15, 505-507.

967. LAUCKNER, W., RETZKE, U., SCHWARTZ, R., and DAUGOTT, E. (1978)
      \Herz-Kreislauf-Veränderungen während der Äthanol-Tokolyse.'
      ['Cardiovascular changes during ethanol tocolysis.'] Zentral-
      blatt für Gynäkologie (Leipzig), 100, 1201-1206.

968. LAUERSEN, N.H., and FUCHS, F. (1973) 'Experience with Shirod-
      kar's operation and postoperative alcohol treatment.' Acta
      Obstetrica et Gynaecologica Scandinavica (Lund), 52, 77-81.

969. LAUERSEN, N.H., RAGHAVAN, K.S., WILSON, K.H., FUCHS, F., and NEI-
      MAN, W.H. (1973) 'Effect of prostaglandin F2 oxytocin, and
      ethanol on the uterus of pregnant baboon.' American Journal
      of Obstetrics and Gynecology, 115, 912.

970. LAUSECKER, C., WITHOFS, L., RITZ, N., and PENNERATH, A. (1976)
      'À propos du syndrome dit "d'alcoolisme foetal."' ['Concerning
      the syndrome called "fetal alcoholism."'] Pédiatrie (Lyons),
      31, 741-747.

971. LEATHEM, J.H. (1966) 'Nutritional effects on hormone produc-
      tion.' Journal of Animal Science, 25 (Supplement), 68-82.

972. LECOMTE, M. (1950) 'Éléments d'hérédopathologie.' ['Elements of
      heredopathology.'] Scalpel (Brussels), 103, 1133-1145.

973. LEE, B.L. (1980) 'Alcohol's effects on the fetus.' The Journal,
      9, 16.

974. LEE, M., and LEICHTER, J. (1980) 'Effect of litter size on the
      physical growth and motivation of the offspring of rats given
      alcohol during gestation.' Growth, 44, 327-335.

975. LEE, M.H., HADDAD, R., and RABE, A. (1980) 'Developmental im-
      pairments in the progeny of rats consuming ethanol during
      pregnancy.' Neurobehavioral Toxicology, 2, 189-198.

976. LEE, M.H., HADDAD, R., RABE, A., and DUMAS, R. (1979) 'Pre-
      weaning learning deficits in progeny of rats consuming eth-
      anol during pregnancy.' Paper presented at the Internation-
      al Society for Developmental Psychobiology, Atlanta,
      Georgia (November).

977. LEE, M.H., RABE, A., HADDAD, R., and DUMAS, R. (1980) 'Develop-
      mental delays in the progeny of rats consuming ethanol during
      pregnancy.' Teratology, 21, 53A (abstract).

978. LEE, M.H.E. (1981) 'Effects on prenatal exposure to ethanol on
      functional development of the rat.' Dissertation Abstracts
      International, 41, 3921B (abstract).

979. LEGRAIN, M. (1895) Dégénérescence social et alcoolisme. [Social
      Degeneration and Alcoholism.] Paris.

980. LEGRAND, A. (1906) Alcoolisme et tuberculose. [Alcoholism and
      Tuberculosis.] Thèse, Lyons.

981. LEIBER, B. (1976) 'Embryopathisches Alkoholismus-Syndrom in
      tausenden Fällen übersehen.' ['Embryopathic alcoholism syn-
      drome reviewed in a thousand cases.'] Medizin, 4, 1365.

982. LEIBER, B. (1977) 'Schwere multiple Missbildungen bei Kindern
      von Alkoholikerinnen nehmen erschreckend zu!' ['Severe
      multiple malformations in children of alcoholic women occur
      shockingly!'] Schleswig-Holsteinisches Ärzteblatt, 2, 89-92.

983. LEIBER, B. (1977) 'Warnhinweis von DOFONOS, das bedeutendste
      teratogene Agens der Gegenwart: Alkohol, erschreckende
      Zunahme von schweren multiplen Missbildungen bei Kindern von
      Trinkerinnen.' ['Warning from DOFONOS; the most current im-
      portant teratogen: Alcohol. An alarming increase in serious
      multiple defects in children of alcoholic mothers.'] Zeit-
      schrift für Allgemeinmedizin (Stuttgart), 53, 2040-2043.

984. LEIBER, B. (1978) 'Alkohol der bedeutsamste missbildungserzeu-
      gende Wirkstoff der Gegenwart. Schwere Mehrfachmissbildungen
      bei Kindern von Trinkerinnen nehmen erschreckend zu. Ein
      Warnhinweis von DOFONOS.' ['Alcohol--currently the most
      significant agent causing malformations. Severe multiple
      abnormalities in children of alcoholics are increasing at an
      alarming rate. A warning from DOFONOS.'] Medizinische
      Monatsschrift für Pharmakologie, 1, 25-26.

985. LEIBER, B. (1978) 'Alkohol-Embryopathie.' ['Alcohol Embryo-
      pathology.'] Deutsche Medizinische Wochenschrift (Stutt-
      gart), 103, 880-881.

986. LEIBER, B., and OLBRICH, G. (1976) 'Embryopathisches Alkohol-
      ismus-Syndrom (Embryopathia alcoholica).' ['Alcohol embryo-
      pathology (embryopathia alcoholica).'] Monatsschrift für
      Kinderheilkunde (Berlin), 124, 43-46.

987. LEICHTER, J., and LEE, M. (1979) 'Effect of maternal ethanol ad-
      ministration on physical growth of the offspring in rats.'
      Growth, 43, 288-297.

988. LEITCH, G.J., and ROSEMOND, R. (1981) 'Failure of zinc supple-
      ment to reverse the teratogenic effects of in utero ethanol.'
      Alcoholism: Clinical and Experimental Research, 5, 159 (ab-
      stract).

989. LEMERE, F., and SMITH, J.W. (1973) 'Alcohol-induced sexual impo-
      tence.' American Journal of Psychiatry, 130, 212-213.

990. LEMOINE, P., HAROUSSEAU, H., BORTERYU, J.P., and MENUET, J.-C.
      (1967) 'Les enfants de parents alcooliques; anomalies obser-
      vées, apropos de 127 cas.' ['The children of alcoholic
      parents; anomalies observed in 127 cases.'] Archives Fran-
      çaises de Pédiatrie, 25, 830-832.

991. LEMOINE, P., HAROUSSEAU, H., BORTERYU, J.-P., and MENUET, J.-C.
      (1968) 'Les enfants de parents alcooliques: Anomalies ob-
      servées à propos de 127 cas.' ['Children of alcoholic
      parents: Anomalies observed in 127 cases.'] Ouest Médicale,
      21, 476-482. (Also published as English translation--Rock-
      ville, Maryland: National Clearinghouse for Alcohol Infor-
      mation, n.d.)

992. LEPAGE, C.P. (1906) Feeblemindedness in Children. Manchester.

993. LEPPÄLUOTO, J., RAPELI, M., VARIS, R., and RANTA, T. (1975) 'Se-
      cretion of anterior pituitary hormones in man: Effect of
      ethyl alcohol.' Acta Physiologica Scandinavica (Stockholm),
      95, 400-406.

994. LESTER, R., and VAN-THIEL, D.H. (1977) 'Gonadal function in
      chronic alcoholic men.' Advances in Experimental Medicine
      and Biology, 85a, 399-414.

995. LESTER, R., and VAN-THIEL, D.H. (1977) 'Gonadal function in
      chronic alcoholic men.' In: Alcohol Intoxication and With-
      drawal--111a: Biological Aspects of Ethanol. Ed. Mil-
      ton M. Gross. New York: Plenum Press, pp. 399-413.

996. LESURE, J.F. (1980) 'Syndrome d'alcoolisme foetal à l'lle de la
      Réunion.' ['Fetal alcohol syndrome in Réunion Island.']
      Nouvelle Presse Médicale (Paris), 9, 1708, 1710.

997. LEVINE, J. (1955) 'The sexual adjustment of alcoholics: A clin-
      ical study of a selected sample.' Quarterly Journal of
      Studies on Alcohol, 16, 675-680.

998. LEWIS, P.J., and BOYLAN, P. (1979) 'Alcohol and fetal
      breathing.' [Letter.] Lancet (London), 1, 388.

999. LIEBER, C.S., SHAW, S., and VAN WAES, L. (1978) 'Alcoholism and
      alcoholic liver injury.' Archives of Pathology and Labora-
      tory Medicine, 102, 393-395.

1000. LIEGEL, J., FABRE, L.F., HOWARD, P.Y., and FARMER, R.W. (1972)
      'Plasma testosterone binding globulin (SBG) in alcoholic sub-
      jects.' Physiologist, 15, 198.

1001. LIKHTANSKII, G.P. (1975) 'Vliyaniye alkogolizma na potomstvo.'
       ['The effect of alcoholism on progeny.'] Vrachebnoe Delo
       (Kiev), 2, 138-139.

1002. LILLY, L.J. (1975) 'Investigations in vitro and in vivo, of the
       effects of disulfiram (antabuse) on human lymphocyte chromo-
       somes.' Toxicology (Amsterdam), 4, 331-340.

1003. LIN, G.W.-J. (1981) 'Effect of ethanol feeding during pregnancy
       on placental transfer of alpha-aminoisobutyric acid in the
       rat.' Life Sciences, 28, 595-601.

1004. LIN, G.W.-J. (1981) 'Effect of ethanol feeding on the urinary his-
       tamine level of the pregnant rat.' Pharmacologist, 23, 218
       (abstract).

1005. LIN, G.W.-J., HAUGEN, E., and LESTER, D. (1978) 'Ethanol and rat
       fetal development.' Federation Proceedings; Federation of
       American Societies for Experimental Biology, 37, 421 (ab-
       stract #1116).

1006. LIN, G.W.-J., and MADDATU, A.P., JR. (1980) 'Effect of ethanol
       feeding during pregnancy on maternal-fetal transfer of ∝-amino-
       isobutyric acid in the rat.' Alcoholism: Clinical and Exper-
       imental Research, 4, 222 (abstract).

1007. LINAKIS, J.G., and CUNNINGHAM, C.L. (1980) 'Behavioral consequen-
       ces of prenatal exposure to alcohol: Effects on discrimina-
       tion, conditioned inhibition, and the transfer of inhibition.'
       Alcoholism: Clinical and Experimental Research, 4, 222 (ab-
       stract).

1008. LINAKIS, J.G., and CUNNINGHAM, C.L. (1980) 'The effects of embry-
       onic exposure to alcohol on learning and inhibition in chicks.'
       Neurobehavioral Toxicology, 2, 243-251.

1009. LINCOLN, D.W. (1973) 'Milk ejection during alcohol anesthesia in
       the rat.' [Letter.] Nature, 243, 227-228.

1010. LINDENSCHMIDT, R.R., and PERSAUD, T.V.N. (1980) 'Effect of
       ethanol and nicotine in the pregnant rat.' Research Commun-
       ications in Chemical Pathology and Pharmacology, 27, 195-198.

1011. LINDHOLM, J., FABRICIUS-BJERRE, N., BAHNSEN, M., BOIESEN, P., BANG-
       STRUP, L., LAU PEDERSEN, M., and HAGEN, C. (1978) 'Pituitary-
       testicular function in patients with chronic alcoholism.'
       European Journal of Clinical Investigation (Berlin), 8, 269-
       272.

1012. LINDHOLM, J., FABRICIUS-BJERRE, N., BAHNSEN, M., BOIESEN, P.,
       HAGEN, C., and CHRISTENSEN, T. (1978) 'Sex steroids and sex-
       hormone binding globulin in males with chronic alcoholism.'
       European Journal of Clinical Investigation (Berlin), 8, 273-
       276.

1013.   LINDOR, E., MC CARTHY, A.-M., and MC RAE, M.G.   (1980)   'Fetal
        alcohol syndrome: A review and case presentation.' JOGN
        Nursing, 9, 222-223, 225-228.

1014.   LINNOILA, M., PRINZ, P.N., WONSOWICZ, C.J., and LEPPÄLUOTO, J.
        (1980)   'Effect of moderate doses of ethanol and phenobarbital
        on pituitary and thyroid hormones and testosterone.' British
        Journal of Addiction, 75, 207-212.

1015.   LIPPICH, F.W.   (1834)   Grundzüge zur Dipsobiostatistik. [Princi-
        ples of Alcohol Biostatistics.] Laibach.

1016.   LIPPMANN, S.   (1980)   'Prenatal alcohol and minimal brain dysfunc-
        tion.' Southern Medical Journal, 73, 1173-1174.

1017.   LIPSON, A.H., YU, J.S., O'HALLORAN, M.T., and WILLIAMS, R.   (1981)
        'Alcohol and phenylketonuria.' [Letter.] Lancet (London), 1,
        717-718.

1018.   LISANSKY, E.S.   (1957)   'Alcoholism in women: Social and psycho-
        logical concomitants. I. Social history data.' Quarterly
        Journal of Studies on Alcohol, 18, 588-623.

1019.   LITKE, L.L.   (1976)   'The effects of various experimental substrates
        on the ventral surface of early chick embryos as observed by
        SEM and TEM.' Anatomical Record, 184, 464.

1020.   LITTLE, R.E.   (1975)   'Alcohol consumption during pregnancy and
        decreased birth weight.' Sc.D Dissertation, Johns Hopkins
        University.

1021.   LITTLE, R.E.   (1976)   'Alcohol consumption during pregnancy as
        reported to the obstetrician and to an independent inter-
        viewer.' Annals of the New York Academy of Sciences, 273,
        588-592.

1022.   LITTLE, R.E.   (1977)   'Moderate alcohol use during pregnancy and
        decreased infant birth weight.' American Journal of Public
        Health, 67, 1154-1156.

1023.   LITTLE, R.E.   (1978)   'History of spontaneous abortion and its
        relation to tobacco and alcohol use in 513 pregnant women.'
        American Journal of Epidemiology, 108, 232 (abstract).

1024.   LITTLE, R.E.   (1978)   'Moderate alcohol use during pregnancy and
        decreased infant birth weight.' Obstetrical and Gynecological
        Survey, 33, 710-712.

1025.   LITTLE, R.E.   (1979)   'Drinking during pregnancy: Implications for
        public health.' Alcohol Health and Research World, 4, 36-42.

1026.   LITTLE, R.E.   (1980)   'Maternal alcohol and tobacco use and nausea
        and vomiting during pregnancy: Relation to infant birthweight.'
        Acta Obstetrica et Gynecologica Scandinavica, 59, 495-497.

1027. LITTLE, R.E. (1980) 'State of the art address: Epidemiologic
           and human studies.' Paper presented at the Fetal Alcohol
           Syndrome Workshop, Seattle, Washington (May 2-4).

1028. LITTLE, R.E. (1981) 'Epidemiologic and experimental studies in
           drinking and pregnancy: The state of the art.' Neurobehav-
           ioral Toxicology and Teratology, 3, 163-167.

1029. LITTLE, R.E. (1981) 'Maternal alcohol use during pregnancy: A
           review.' In: Fetal Alcohol Syndrome. Volume 2: Human
           Studies. Ed. E.L. Abel. Boca Raton, Florida: CRC Press
           (in press).

1030. LITTLE, R.E., GRATHWOHL, H.L., STREISSGUTH, A.P., and MC INTYRE, C.
           (1981) 'Public awareness and knowledge about the risks of
           drinking during pregnancy in Multnomah County, Oregon.' Amer-
           ican Journal of Public Health, 71, 312-314.

1031. LITTLE, R.E., and HOOK, E. (1979) 'Maternal alcohol and tobacco
           consumption associated with nausea and vomiting during
           pregnancy.' Acta Obstetrica et Gynecologia Scandinavica
           (Lund), 58, 15-17.

1032. LITTLE, R.E., MOORE, D.E., GUZINSKI, G.M., and PEREZ, A. (1980)
           'Absence of effect of exogenous estradiol on alcohol con-
           sumption in women.' Substance and Alcohol Actions/Misuse, 1,
           551-556.

1033. LITTLE, R.E., and QUINN, S. (1979) 'Alcohol and pregnancy.'
           [Letter.] Alcoholism: Clinical and Experimental Research,
           3, 92.

1034. LITTLE, R.E., and SCHULTZ, F. (1974) 'Drinking behavior in 156
           pregnant women.' Paper presented at the North American Con-
           gress on Alcohol and Drug Problems, San Francisco, California.

1035. LITTLE, R.E., SCHULTZ, F.A., and MANDELL, W. (1976) 'Drinking
           during pregnancy.' Journal of Studies on Alcohol, 37, 375-
           379.

1036. LITTLE, R.E., and STREISSGUTH, A.P. (1978) "Drinking during
           pregnancy in alcoholic women.' Alcohol: Clinical and Exper-
           imental Research, 2, 179-183.

1037. LITTLE, R.E., and STREISSGUTH, A.P. (1978) 'Drug use in pregnant
           alcoholic women.' Paper presented at the National Drug Abuse
           Conference, Seattle, Washington.

1038. LITTLE, R.E., and STREISSGUTH, A.P. (1981) 'Effects of alcohol on
           the fetus: Impact and prevention.' Canadian Medical Assoc-
           iation Journal, 125, 159-164.

1039. LITTLE, R.E., STREISSGUTH, A.P., BARR, H.M., and HERMAN, C.S.
           (1980) 'Decreased birth weight in infants of alcoholic women
           who abstained during pregnancy.' Journal of Pediatrics, 96,
           974-977.

1040. LITTLE, R.E., STREISSGUTH, A.P., and GUZINSKI, G.M. (1980) 'Prevention of fetal alcohol syndrome: A model program.' Alcoholism: Clinical and Experimental Research, 4, 185-189.

1041. LITTLE, R.E., STREISSGUTH, A.P., and PAGE, E. (1979) 'Techniques for recruiting special types of persons for research: Pitfalls and successes in enlisting recovered alcoholic women.' Public Health Reports, 94, 332-335.

1042. LITTLE, R.E., STREISSGUTH, A.P., WOODELL, S., and NORDEN, R. (1979) 'Birthweight of infants born to recovered alcoholic women.' Alcoholism: Clinical and Experimental Research, 3, 184 (abstract).

1043. LKKEN, P. (1981) 'Fetal alcohol syndrome.' Nor Tannlaegeforen Tidschrift, 91, 204-206.

1044. LLOYD, C.W., and WILLIAMS, R.H. (1948) 'Endocrine changes associated with Laennec's cirrhosis of the liver.' American Journal of Medicine, 4, 315-330.

1045. LOCHRY, E.A., and RILEY, E.P. (1980) 'Effects of prenatal alcohol on learning and retention in the rat.' Alcoholism: Clinical and Experimental Research, 4, 222 (abstract).

1046. LOCHRY, E.A., and RILEY, E.P. (1980) 'Retention of passive avoidance and T-maze escape in rats exposed to alcohol prenatally.' Neurobehavioral Toxicology, 2, 107-115.

1047. LOCHRY, E.A., SHAPIRO, N.R., and RILEY, E.P. (1979) 'Operant behavior in rats exposed to alcohol prenatally.' Alcoholism: Clinical and Experimental Research, 3, 185 (abstract).

1048. LOCHRY, E.A., SHAPIRO, N.R., and RILEY, E.P. (1980) 'Growth deficits in rats exposed to alcohol in utero.' Journal of Studies on Alcohol, 41, 1031-1039.

1049. LOIODICE, G., FORTUNA, G., GUIDETTI, A., RIA, N., and D'ELIA, R. (1975) 'Considerazioni cliniche intorno a du casi di malformazioni congenite in bambine nati da madri affette da alcoolismo cronico (primi casi Italiani).' ['Clinical notes on two cases of congenital deformity in children born of chronic alcoholic mothers (first Italian cases).'] Minerva Pediatrica (Torino), 27, 1891-1893.

1050. LOIODICE, G., PRUSEK, W., and SCIANARO, L. (1975) 'Zespoł płodu alkoholizowanego-spotrzezenia własne.' [Fetal alcohol syndrome: Case reports.'] Polski Tygodnik Lekarski (Warsaw), 33, 1857-1858.

1051. LOOSLI, R., LOUSTALOT, P., SCHALCH, W.R., SIEVERS, K., and STENGER, E.G. (1964) 'Joint study in teratogenicity research: Preliminary communication.' Proceedings of the European's Society for the Study of Drug Toxicity. Volume 4: Some Factors Affecting Drug Toxicity. New York: Excerpta Medica, p. 214.

1052. LOPEZ, R., and MONTOYA, M.F. (1971) 'Abnormal bone marrow mor-
         phology in the premature infant associated with maternal
         alcohol infusion.' Journal of Pediatrics, 79, 1008-1010.

1053. LÖSER, H. (1977) 'Alkoholembryopathie--ein häufiges Fehlbildungs-
         syndrom.' [Alcohol embryopathy--a frequent malformation syn-
         drome.'] Hippokrates (Stuttgart), 48, 272-273.

1054. LÖSER, H., and MAJEWSKI, F. (1977) 'Type and frequency of car-
         diac defects in embryofetal alcohol syndrome: Report of 16
         cases.' British Heart Journal (London), 39, 1374-1379.

1055. LÖSER, H., MAJEWSKI, F., APITZ, J., and BIERICH, J. R. (1975)
         'Kardiovaskuläre Fehlbildungen bei fetalem Alkohol-Syndrom.'
         ['Cardiovascular defects in fetal alcohol syndrome.'] Zeit-
         schrift für Kardiologie, Supplementum (Darmstadt), 2, 91.

1056. LÖSER, H., MAJEWSKI, F., APITZ, J., and BIERICH, J.R. (1976)
         'Kardiovaskuläre Fehlbildungen bei embryofetalem Alkohol-
         Syndrom.' ['Cardiovascular defects in fetal alcohol syn-
         drome.'] Klinische Pädiatrie (Stuttgart), 188, 233-240.

1057. LOWRY, R.B. (1977) 'The Klippel-Feil anomalad as part of the
         fetal alcohol syndrome.' Teratology, 16, 53-56.

1058. LOX, C.D., MESSIHA, F., and HEINE, M.W. (1981) 'The influence of
         ethanol and oral contraceptives on reproductive physiology in
         the female rat.' Fertility and Sterility, 35 (Supplement),
         241 (abstract).

1059. LOX, C.D., MESSIHA, F., HEINE, M.W., BENSON, B., and MISENHIMER,
         G.R. (1980) 'Ethanol and reproductive function in the female
         rat.' Pharmacology, Biochemistry, and Behavior, 12, 326.

1060. LOX, C.D., PEDDICORD, O., HEINE, M.W., and MESSIHA, F.S. (1978)
         'The influence of chronic long term alcohol abuse on testos-
         terone secretion in men and rats.' Proceedings of the Western
         Pharmacology Society, 21, 299-302.

1061. LUI, A. (1900) 'Eredita ed alcoolismo.' ['Heredity and alco-
         holism.'] Annali di Neurologia, 18, 36.

1062. LUKE, B. (1977) 'Maternal alcoholism and fetal alcoholism.'
         American Journal of Nursing, 77, 1924-1926.

1063. LUMPKIN, J.R., BAKER, F.J., II, and FRANASZEK, F.B. (1979) 'Alco-
         holic ketoacidosis in a pregnant woman.' Journal of the Amer-
         ican College of Emergency Physicians, 8, 21-23.

1064. LUUKKANINEN, T., VAISTO, L., and JARVINEN, P.A. (1967) 'The ef-
         fect of oral intake of ethyl alcohol on the activity of the
         pregnant human uterus.' Acta Obstetrica et Gynecologica
         Scandinavica (Lund), 46 486-493.

1065. LYNN, J.M. (1970) 'Intravenous alcohol infusion for premature labor.' Journal of the American Osteopathic Association, 70, 167-170.

1066. LYONS, J.P., RUSSELL, M., and BROWN, J. (1980) 'Computer-aided alcoholism diagnosis in ob-gyn settings.' Alcoholism: Clinical and Experimental Research, 4, 222 (abstract).

1067. LYUBIMOV, B.I., and SMOLNIKOVA, N.M. (1981) 'The effect of psychotropic drugs and alcohol on offspring development.' In: Eighth International Congress of Pharmacology. Tokyo: Japanese Pharmacological Society and Science Council of Japan (July 19-24), p. 121 (abstract).

1068. LYUBIMOV, B.I., SMOLNIKOVA, N.M., STREKALOVA, S.N., KUROCHKIN, I.G., MITROFANOV, V.S., PORFIRIEVA, R.P., MARKIN, V.A., and SHAROV, P.A. (1979) 'Preclinical trials of the new tranquilizer phenazepam safety.' Farmakologiia i Toksikologiia, 42, 464-467.

1069. LYUBIMOV, B.I., SMOLNIKOVA, N.M., STREKALOVA, S.N., and YAVORSKII, A.N. (1979) "Vliyaniye karbidina na polovyye zhelezy krys pri khronicheskom vozdeistvii etanola.' ['Effect of carbidine on the gonads of rats during chronic alcohol poisoning.] Byulleten Eksperimental noi Biologii Meditsiny, 87, 155-158.

M

1070. MC CONNELL, H. (1979) 'Goodwin draws bead on some "poppycock": A sceptic's approach to alcohol.' The Journal, 8, 16.

1071. MC CONNELL, H. (1981) 'Obs/gyne chiefs need alert to FAS.' The Journal, 10, 2 (June 1).

1072. MC DANIEL, W.H. (1883) 'The effect of alcohol upon the foetus through the blood of the mother.' Maryland State Medical Journal, 10, 39-40.

1073. MC DONALD, J.S. (1977) 'Preanesthetic and intrapartal medications.' Clinical Obstetrics and Gynecology, 20, 447-459.

1074. MAC DONALD. R.N. (1978) Starting a Healthy Family. Newton, Massachusetts: Education Development Center.

1075. MAC DOWELL, E.C. (1915) 'Parental alcoholism and mental ability.' Science, 42, 680.

1076. MAC DOWELL, E.C. (1922) 'Alcohol and white rats; a study of fertility.' Proceedings of the Society for Experimental Biology and Medicine, 19, 69-71.

1077. MAC DOWELL, E.C. (1922) 'Experiments with alcohol and white rats.' American Naturalist, 56, 289-311.

1078. MAC DOWELL, E.C. (1923) 'Alcoholism and the behavior of white rats. II. The maze behavior of treated rats and their offspring.' Journal of Experimental Zoology, 37, 417-456.

1079. MAC DOWELL, E.C., and LORD, E.M. (1927) 'Reproduction in alcoholic mice. I. Treated females. A study of the influence of alcohol on ovarian activity, prenatal mortality, and sex ratio.' [Wilhelm] Roux's Archives of Developmental Biology, 109, 549-581.

1080. MAC DOWELL, E.C., LORD, E.M., and MAC DOWELL, C.H. (1926) 'Heavy alcoholization and prenatal morality in mice.' Proceedings of the Society for Experimental Biology and Medicine, 23, 652-654.

1081. MAC DOWELL, E.C., and VICARI, E.M. (1917) 'On the growth and fecundity of alcoholized rats.' Proceedings of the National Academy of Sciences of the United States of America, 3, 577-579.

1082. MAC DOWELL, E.C., and VICARI, E.M. (1921) 'Alcoholism and the behavior of white rats. I. The influence of alcoholic grand-parents upon maze behavior.' Journal of Experimental Zoology, 33, 209-291.

1083. MC FALLS, J.A., JR. (1979) 'Alcoholism.' In: Psychopathology and Subfecundity. Ed. J.A. Mc Falls, Jr. New York: Aca-demic.

1084. MC ILROY, A.L. (1923) 'The influence of alcohol and alcoholism upon antenatal and infant life.' British Journal of Inebriety, 21, 39-42.

1085. MC INTYRE, C.E. (1980) 'Evaluating prevention and education: Fetal alcohol syndrome.' Paper presented at the National Council on Alcohol Conference, Seattle, Washington.

1086. MC LACHLAN, J.A., NEWBOLD, R.R., and BULLOCK, B.C. (1980) 'Long-term effects on the female mouse genital tract associated with prenatal exposure to diethylstilbestrol.' Cancer Research, 40, 3988-3999.

1087. MC LAUGHLIN, J., JR., MARLIAC, J.-P., VERRETT, M.J., MUTCHLER, M.K., and FITZHUGH, O.G. (1963) 'The injection of chemicals into the yolk sac of fertile eggs prior to incubation as a toxicity test.' Toxicology and Applied Pharmacology, 5, 760-771.

1088. MC LAUGHLIN, J., JR., MARLIAC, J.-P., VERRETT, J., MUTCHLER, M.K., and FITZHUGH, O.G. (1964) 'Toxicity of fourteen volatile chemicals as measured by the chick embryo method.' American Industrial Hygiene Association, 25, 282-284.

1089. MC LAUGHLIN, J., JR., and MUTCHLER, M.K. (1962) 'Toxicity of some chemicals measured by injection into chicken eggs.' Feder-ation Proceedings, 21, 450 (abstract).

1090. MACMILLAN, K.L. (1973) 'The effect of benzyl alcohol on the oestrous cycle of cattle.' Australian Veterinary Journal (Sydney), 49, 267-268.

1091. MACMILLAN, K.L., HART, N.L., WATSON, J.D., and SMITH, J.F. (1974) 'Effects of benzyl alcohol on the bovine oestrous cycle and subsequent fertility.' Theriogenology, 1, 1-5.

1092. MC MILLEN, M. (1980) 'Alcohol education: Fetal alcohol syn-drome.' Oklahoma Nurse, 25, 5.

1093. MC NALL, L.K., and COLLEA, J. (1978) 'Environmental influences on embryonic and fetal development.' Current Practice Obstet-rical Gynecological Nursing, 2, 67-90.

1094. MC NAMEE, B., GRANT, J., RATCLIFFE, J., RATCLIFFE, W. and OLIVER, J.
       (1979) 'Lack of effect of alcohol on pituitary-gonadal hor-
       mones in women.' British Journal of Addiction (Edinburgh), 74,
       316-317.

1095. MAC NICHOLL, T.A. (1905) 'A study of the effects of alcohol on
       school children.' Quarterly Journal of Inebriety, 27, 113-
       117.

1096. MAC NISH, R. (1835) The Anatomy of Drunkenness. 5th Glasgow
       edition. New York: Appleton.

1097. MAGNAN, V., and FILLINGER, A. (1913) 'Alcoolisme et degénér-
       escence.' ['Alcoholism and degeneration.'] Revue d'Hygiene
       (Paris), 35, 266-281.

1098. MAIRET, A., and COMBEMALE, F. (1888) 'Influence degénérative de
       l'alcool sur la descendance.' ['Degenerative influence of
       alcohol on the offspring.'] Recherches Experimentelles
       Comptes Rendus des Séances de l'Académie des Sciences, 106,
       667.

1099. MAJDECKI, T. (1979) 'Embriopatia alkoholowa--nowy zespól choro-
       bowy.' ['Alcohol embryopathy--A new syndrome.'] Neurologia
       i Neurochirurgia Polska, 13, 665-669.

1100. MAJDECKI, T., BESKID, M., SKLADZINSKI, J., and MARCINIAK, M.
       (1976) 'Effect of ethanol application during pregnancy on
       the electron microscopic image of a newborn brain.' Materia
       Medica Polona (Warsaw), 8, 365-370.

1101. MAJEWSKI, F. (1977) 'Über einige durch teratogene Noxen indu-
       zierte Fehlbildungen.' ['On certain embryopathies induced by
       teratogenic noxae.'] Monatschrift für Kinderheilkunde (Ber-
       lin), 125, 609-620.

1102. MAJEWSKI, F. (1978) 'Über schädigende Einflüsse des Alkohols auf
       die Nachkommen.' ['The damaging effects of alcohol on off-
       spring.'] Nervenarzt (Berlin), 49, 410-416.

1103. MAJEWSKI, F. (1978) 'Untersuchungen zur Alkohol-Embryopathie.'
       ['Investigations in alcohol embryopathy.'] Fortschritte der
       Medizin (Munich), 96, 2207-2213.

1104. MAJEWSKI, F. (1979) 'Die Alkoholembryopathie: Fakten und Hypo-
       thesen.' ['Alcoholic embryopathology: Facts and hypotheses.']
       Ergebnisse Internal Medizinische Kinderheilkunke 43, 1-55.

1105. MAJEWSKI, F. (1980) 'Alcohol embryopathy and diabetic fetopathy
       in the same newborn.' European Journal of Pediatrics (in
       press).

1106. MAJEWSKI, F. (1980) 'On the pathogenesis of alcohol embryopathy:
       Facts and speculations.' Paper presented at the Fetal Alcohol
       Syndrome Workshop, Seattle, Washington (May 2-4).

1107. MAJEWSKI, F. (1980) Untersuchungen zur Alkoholembryopathie.
       [Studies on Alcohol Embryopathy.] Stuttgart and New York:
       Thieme.

1108. MAJEWSKI, F. (1980) 'Variations in face and growth with in-
       creasing age (clinical studies from Germany).' Paper pre-
       sented at the Fetal Alcohol Syndrome Workshop, Seattle,
       Washington (May 2-4).

1109. MAJEWSKI, F. (1981) 'Alcohol embryopathy: Some facts and specu-
       lations about pathogenesis.' Neurobehavioral Toxicology and
       Teratology, 3, 129-144.

1110. MAJEWSKI, F., and BIERICH, J.R. (1979) 'Auxological and clinical
       findings in the alcohol embryopathy: Experience with 76
       patients.' Acta Medica Scandinavica, 206, 413-423.

1111. MAJEWSKI, F., BIERICH, J.R., LÖSER, H., MICHAELIS, R., LEIBER, B.,
       and BETTECKEN, F. (1976) 'Zur Klinik und Pathogenese der
       Alkohol-Embryopathie; Bericht über 68 Fälle.' ['Clinical
       aspects and pathogenesis of alcohol embryopathy: A report of
       68 cases.'] Münchener Medizinische Wochenschrift (Munich),
       118, 1635-1642.

1112. MAJEWSKI, F., BIERICH, J.R., and MICHAELIS, R. (1976) 'Diagnose:
       Alkohol Embryopathie.' ['Diagnosis: Alcohol embryopath-
       ology.'] Deutsches Ärzteblatt, 17, 1133-1136.

1113. MAJEWSKI, F., BIERICH, J.R., and MICHAELIS, R. (1977) 'Diagnose:
       Alkoholembryopathie.' ['Diagnosis: Alcohol embryopathy.']
       Jahrgang/Heft, 17, 1133-1136.

1114. MAJEWSKI, F., BIERICH, J.R., MICHAELIS, R., LÖSER, H., and LEIB-
       ER, B. (1977) 'Über die Alkohol-Embryopathie, eine häufige
       intrauterine Schädigung.' ['On alcohol embryopathy, a fre-
       quent source of intrauterine damage.'] Monatsschrift für
       Kinderheilkunde (Berlin), 125, 445-446.

1115. MAJEWSKI, F., BIERICH, J.R., and SEIDENBERG, J. (1978) 'Zur
       Häufigkeit und Pathogenese des Alkoholembryopathie.' ['On
       the frequency and pathology of alcohol embryopathy.'] Monats-
       schrift für Kinderheilkunde (Berlin), 126, 284-285.

1116. MAJEWSKI, F., FISCHBACH, H., PFEIFFER, J., and BIERICH, J.R.
       (1978) 'Zur Frage des Interruptio bei Alkoholkranken Frauen.'
       ['Interruption of pregnancy in alcoholic women.'] Deutsche
       Medizinische Wochenschrift (Stuttgart), 103, 895-898.

1117. MAJEWSKI, F., and GOECKE, T. (1981) 'Alcohol embryopathy:
       Studies in Germany.' In: Fetal Alcohol Syndrome. Volume 2:
       Human Studies. Ed. E.L. Abel. Boca Raton, Florida: CRC
       Press (in press).

1118. MAJEWSKI, F., NOTHJUNGE, J., and BIERICH, J.R. (1979) 'Alcohol
       embryopathy and diabetic fetopathy in the same newborn.'
       Helvetica Paediatrica Acta (Basel), 34, 135-139.

1119. MALAKHORSKIJI, V.G., and PROZOROVSKI, V.B. (1975) 'Behavioral dis-
       order in the progeny of rat subjected to chronic action of al-
       cohol.' Farmakologiia i Toksikologiia (Moscow), 38, 88-90.

1120. MALATESTA, V.J. (1978) 'The effects of alcohol on ejaculation
       latency in human males.' Ph.D. Thesis, University of Georgia.

1121. MALATESTA, V.J. POLLACK, R.H., and CROTTY, T.D. (1979) 'Alcohol
       effects on the orgasmic response in human females.' Paper
       presented at the Annual Meeting of the Psychonomic Society,
       Phoenix, Arizona (November).

1122. MALATESTA, V.J., POLLACK, R.H., WILBANKS, W.A., and ADAMS, H.E.
       (1979) 'Alcohol effects on the orgasmic-ejaculatory response
       in human males.' Journal of Sex Research, 15, 101-107.

1123. MALAVIYA, B., SINGH, M.M., CHANDRA, H., and DASGUPTA, P.R. (1976)
       'Fetal resorption in rats following intrauterine instillation
       of alcohol.' Indian Journal of Experimental Biology, 14, 316.

1124. MALONEY, S.K., BAST, R.J., and O'GORMAN, P. (1980) 'Perspectives
       on prevention of fetal alcohol effects.' Neurobehavioral
       Toxicology, 2, 271-276.

1125. MANDERS, D., and SINCLAIR, E. (1980) 'Public education concerning
       the fetal alcohol syndrome.' Paper presented at the National
       Council on Alcohol Conference, Seattle, Washington.

1126. MANKAD, V.N., and CHOKSI, R.M. (1976) 'The fetal alcohol syn-
       drome.' [Letter.] Journal of the American Medical Assoc-
       iation, 236, 1114.

1127. MANKU, M.S., HORROBIN, D.F., and OKA, M. (1979) 'Differential
       regulation of the formation of prostaglandins and related sub-
       stances from arachidonic acid and from dihomogammalinoleic
       acid. I. Effects of ethanol.' Prostaglandins and Medicine,
       3, 119-128.

1128. MANN, L.I., BHAKTHAVATHSALAN, A., LIU, M., and MAKOWSKI, P. (1975)
       'Effect of alcohol on fetal cerebral function and metabolism.'
       American Journal of Obstetrics and Gynecology, 122, 845-851.

1129. MANN, L.I., BHAKTHAVATHSALAN, A., LIU, M., and MAKOWSKI, P. (1975)
       'Placental transport of alcohol and its effect on maternal and
       fetal acid-base balance.' American Journal of Obstetrics and
       Gynecology, 122, 837-844.

1130. MANN, T. (1968) 'Effects of pharmacological agents on male sexual
       functions.' Journal of Reproduction and Fertility (Oxford), 4
       (Supplement), 101-114.

1131.   MANTELL, C.D., and LIGGINS, G.C.   (1970)   'The effect of ethanol
        on the myometrial response to oxytocin in women at term.'
        Journal of Obstetrics and Gynecology of the British Common-
        wealth, 77, 976-981.

1132.   MANZKE, H., and GROSSE, F.R.   (1975)   'Inkomplettes und Komplettes
        des Alkohol-Syndrom: Bei drei Kindern einer Trinkerin.'   ['In-
        complete and complete alcohol syndrome: Three children of a
        drinker.']   Medizinische Welt (Stuttgart), 26, 709-712.

1133.   MANZKE, H., and SPRETER VON KREUDENSTEIN, P.   (1979)   'Embryofetales
        Alkoholsyndrom.'   ['Fetal alcohol syndrome.']   Suchtgefahren
        (Hamburg), 25, 157-166.

1134.   MARCINIAK, M., MAJDECKI, T., OPAŁKA, S., and DĄMBSKA, M.   (1974)
        'Wpływ etanolu na rozwijający się mózg psa (dzliałanie drogą
        transłożyskową i pokarmową).'   ['Effect of ethanol on devel-
        oping dog brain: Transplacental and alimentary action.']
        Neuropatologia Polska, 12, 27-33.

1135.   MARGOLIN, F.G.   (1977)   'Fetal alcohol syndrome: Report of a case.'
        Journal of the American Osteopathic Association, 77, 50-52.

1136.   MARLATT, G.A., DEMMING, B., and REID, J.B.   (1973)   'Loss of con-
        trol drinking in alcoholics: An experimental analogue.'
        Journal of Abnormal Psychology, 81, 233-241.

1137.   MAROTEAUX, P.   (1960)   'Alcohol et descendance.'   ['Alcohol and
        offspring.']   11e Journées Etude sur le Nouveaune.   Paris,
        Ecole de Puericulture.

1138.   MARTIN, D.C., BARR, H.M., and STREISSGUTH, A.P.   (1980)   'Birth
        weight, birth length, and head circumference related to mater-
        nal alcohol, nicotine and caffeine use during pregnancy.'
        Teratology, 21, 54A (abstract).

1139.   MARTIN, D.C., MARTIN, J.C., STREISSGUTH, A.P., and LUND, C.A.
        (1979)   'Sucking frequency and amplitude in newborns as a
        function of maternal drinking and smoking.'   In: Currents
        in Alcoholism.   Volume 5: Biomedical Issues and Clinical
        Effects of Alcoholism.   Ed. Marc Galanter.   New York: Grune
        and Stratton, pp. 359-366.

1140.   MARTIN, D.C., STREISSGUTH, A.P., and BARR, H.M.   (1980)   'The con-
        tributions of maternal alcohol, nicotine, and caffeine use to
        infant birth weight, birth length, and head circumference.'
        Teratology (in press).

1141.   MARTIN, J.C.   (1976)   'Operant performance of rat offspring on
        appetitive and noxious schedules following maternal ethanol
        exposure.'   Teratology, 13, 30A (abstract).

1142.   MARTIN, J.C.   (1977)   'Offspring survival, development and operant
        performance following maternal ethanol administration.'
        Paper presented at the Fetal Alcohol Syndrome Workshop,
        San Diego, California.

1143. MARTIN, J.C.   (1977)   'The fetal alcohol syndrome: Recent find-
       ings.' Alcohol Health and Research World, 2, 8-12.

1144. MARTIN, J.C.   (1977)   'Maternal alcohol ingestion and cigarette
       smoking and their effects upon newborn conditioning.'
       Alcoholism: Clinical and Experimental Research, 1, 243-247.

1145. MARTIN, J.C.   (1977)   'Offspring survival, development, and operant
       performance following maternal ethanol consumption.' NIAAA-
       sponsored Fetal Alcohol Syndrome Workshop, San Diego, Cali-
       fornia.

1146. MARTIN, J.C., MARTIN, D.C., and DAY-PFEIFFER, H.   (1980)   'The
       interactive effects of maternal nicotine and alcohol on rat
       offspring growth, development and activity.' Teratology,
       21, 77A (abstract).

1147. MARTIN, J.C., MARTIN, D.C., LUND, C.A., and STREISSGUTH, A.P.
       (1977)   'Maternal alcohol ingestion and cigarette smoking
       and their effects on newborn conditioning.' Alcoholism:
       Clinical and Experimental Research, 1, 243-247.

1148. MARTIN, J.C., MARTIN, D.C., RADOW, B., and SIGMAN, G.   (1978)
       'Blood alcohol level and caloric intake in the gravid rat as
       a function of diurnal period, trimester, and vehicle.'
       Pharmacology, Biochemistry, and Behavior, 8, 421-427.

1149. MARTIN, J.C., MARTIN, D.C., SIGMAN, P., and RADOW, B.   (1977)
       'Offspring survival, development, and operant performance
       following maternal ethanol consumption.' Developmental
       Psychobiology, 10, 435-445.

1150. MARTIN, J.C., MARTIN, D.C., SIGMAN, G., and RADOW, B.   (1978)
       'Maternal ethanol consumption and hyperactivity in cross-
       fostered offspring.' Physiological Psychology, 6, 362-365.

1151. MARTIN-BOYCE, A., SCHWARTZ, D., DREYFUS, J., and SCHNEEGANS, P.
       (1978)   'Biochemical and haematological markers of alcohol
       intake.' Lancet (London), 2, 529.

1152. MASTERS, W.H., and JOHNSON, V.E.   (1966)   Human Sexual Response.
       Boston: Little, Brown, and Company, pp. 267-268.

1153. MASTERS, W.H., and JOHNSON, V.E.   (1970)   Human Sexual Inadequacy.
       Boston: Little, Brown, and Company.

1154. MASUR, J.   (1980)   'Maternal alcohol use and clinical condition of
       the newborn: A prospective study in Brazil.' Paper presented
       at the Fetal Alcohol Syndrome Workshop, Seattle, Washington
       (May 2-4).

1155. MATHEWS, D., and JAMISON, S.   (1980)   'Effects of ethanol consump-
       tion on maternal behavior in the female rat.' Eastern Con-
       ference of Reproductive Behavior, New York (June 22-25).

1156. MATHINOS, P. (1980) 'Review of physical anomalies resulting from
       prenatal alcohol exposure.' Paper presented at the meeting
       of the International Society for Developmental Psychobiology,
       Cincinnati (November 8).

1157. MATSUNAGA, E., and SHIOTA, K. (1977) 'Holoprosencephaly in
       human embryos: Epidemiologic studies of 150 cases.' Tera-
       tology, 16, 261-272.

1158. MATSUNAGA, E., and SHIOTA, K. (1980) 'Search for maternal factors
       associated with malformed human embryos: A prospective study.'
       Teratology, 21, 323-331.

1159. MATZDORF, F. (1942) 'Ist der Verlauf der Alkoholkurve in der
       Milch stillender Frauen von der Milchbildung und Milchaus-
       scheidung abhängig?' ['Is the course of the alcohol curve
       in the milk of nursing women dependent on the formation and
       extrusion of milk?'] Klinische Wochenschrift (Berlin), 21,
       131.

1160. MAU, G. (1974) 'Nahrungs- und Genussmittelkonsum in der
       Schwangerschaft und seine Auswirkungen auf perinatale Sterb-
       lichkeit, Frühgeburtlichkeit und andere perinatale Faktoren.'
       ['Diet and average consumption in pregnancy and its effects
       on perinatal mortality, premature birth, and other perinatal
       factors.'] Monatsschrift für Kinderheilkunde, 122, 539-540.

1161. MAU, G. (1980) 'Moderate alcohol consumption during pregnancy
       and child development.' European Journal of Pediatrics,
       133, 233-238.

1162. MAU, G. (1980) 'Premature birth and intrauterine growth retard-
       ation: Evaluation of the risk caused by preexistent mater-
       nal factors.' Medizinische Welt, 31, 237-240.

1163. MAU, G., and NETTER, P. (1974) 'Kaffee- und Alkoholkonsum--
       Risikofactoren in der Schwangerschaft?' ['Coffee and alco-
       hol consumption--Risk factors in pregnancy?'] Geburtshilfe
       und Frauenheilkunde (Stuttgart), 34, 1018-1022.

1164. MAUGH, T.H., III. (1979) 'Alcohol briefing.' Science, 214,
       643-644.

1165. MAYKUT, M.O. (1979) 'Consequences of prenatal maternal alcohol
       exposure including the fetal alcohol syndrome.' Progress in
       Neuro-Psychopharmacology, 3, 465-481.

1166. MAYO, E.E. (1979) 'The relationship between self-concept vari-
       ables and sexual preferences among male alcoholics and male
       non-alcoholics.' Ph.D. dissertation, University of Colorado
       at Boulder.

1167. MEANS, L.W., POTTS, F.L., and CLIETT, C.E. (1981) 'Effects of
       housing density, restraint, and shock on alcohol consumption
       in rats exposed to alcohol in utero.' Alcoholism: Clinical
       and Experimental Research, 5, 349 (abstract).

1168. MEDHUS, A.   (1975)   'Venereal diseases among female alcoholics.'
       Scandinavian Journal of Social Medicine, 3, 29.

1169. MEDICAL WORLD NEWS.   (1969)   'Does drinking peril late-stage
       fetus?' 10, 16.

1170. MEDICAL WORLD NEWS.   (1970)   'Alcohol and pregnancy: Round
       three.' 11, 24.

1171. MEDICAL WORLD NEWS.   (1977)   'Drinking and pregnancy: The govern-
       ment is concerned.' April 18, pp. 26-27.

1172. MEDICAL WORLD NEWS.   (1977)   'Must pregnant women stop drinking?'
       June 27, pp. 9-10.

1173. MEDICAL WORLD NEWS.   (1977)   'Alcohol indicated as strong tera-
       togen.' September 17, pp. 14-15.

1174. MEDICAL WORLD NEWS.   (1977)   'FDA wants birth defect warning on
       booze bottles and more PPIs.' November 14, p. 16.

1175. MEDICAL WORLD NEWS.   (1978)   'Prenatal binge yields healthy
       twins.' December 25, p. 23.

1176. MEDICAL WORLD NEWS.   (1979)   'Alcohol exposure goes to the bones
       of developing fetus.' August 6, pp. 9, 13.

1177. MEHRA, K.S., RAGHVAN, P.K.D., and CHAUDHURY, R.R.   (1970)   'Effect
       of intravenous alcohol on premature labour.' Indian Journal
       of Gynaecology and Obstetrics, 8, 160-161.

1178. MENA, M.R., ALBORNOZ, C.V., PUENTE, M.C., and MORENO, C.   (1980)
       'Síndrome fetal alcohólico: Estudio de 19 casos clínicos.'
       ['Fetal alcohol syndrome: A study of 19 clinical cases.']
       Revista Chilena de Pediatria, 51, 414-423.

1179. MENDELSON, J.H.   (1978)   'The fetal alcohol syndrome.' [Letter.]
       New England Journal of Medicine, 299, 556.

1180. MENDELSON, J.H.   (1979)   'The fetal alcohol syndrome.' Advances
       in Alcoholism, 1, 1-4.

1181. MENDELSON, J.H.   (1981)   'Alcohol effects on sexual behavior and
       hormonal function.' Paper presented at the World Psychiatric
       Meeting, New York (October 31-November 1).

1182. MENDELSON, J.H., ELLINGBOE, J., and MELLO, N.K.   (1978)   'Effects
       of alcohol on plasma testosterone and luteinizing hormone
       levels.' Alcoholism: Clinical and Experimental Research,
       2, 255-258.

1183.   MENDELSON, J.H., ELLINGBOE, J., and MELLO, N.K. (1980) 'Ethanol
        induced alterations in pituitary gonadal hormones in human
        males.' In: Biological Effects of Alcohol: Proceedings
        of the International Symposium on Biological Research in
        Alcoholism, Zurich, Switzerland (June, 1978). Ed. H. Beg-
        leiter. New York and London: Plenum Press, pp. 485-497.

1184.   MENDELSON, J.H., and MELLO, N.K. (1974) 'Alcohol, aggression,
        and androgens.' Research Publications, Association for
        Research in Nervous and Mental Disorders, 52, 225-247.

1185.   MENDELSON, J.H., MELLO, N.K., and ELLINGBOE, J. (1977) 'Effects
        of acute alcohol intake on pituitary-gonadal hormones in
        normal human males.' Journal of Pharmacology and Exper-
        imental Therapeutics, 202, 676-682.

1186.   MENDELSON, J.H., MELLO, N.K., and ELLINGBOE, J. (1978) 'Effects
        of alcohol on pituitary-gonadal hormones, sexual function,
        and aggression in human males.' In: Psychopharmacology:
        A Generation of Progress. Ed. M.A. Lipton, A. DiMascio, and
        K.F. Killam. New York: Raven, pp. 1677-1692.

1187.   MENDELSON, J.H., MELLO, N.K., and ELLINGBOE, J. (1981) 'Acute
        alcohol intake and pituitary gonadal hormones in normal
        human females.' Journal Pharmacology and Experimental
        Therapeutics, 218, 23-26.

1188.   MENDELSON, R., and HUBER, A.M. (1979) 'Maternal alcohol con-
        sumption: Effect of alcohol on trace element deposition in
        the fetus.' Alcoholism: Clinical and Experimental Research,
        3, 186 (abstract).

1189.   MENDELSON, R., and HUBER, A.M. (1979) 'The effect of chronic
        and acute alcohol administration on trace element uptake by
        rats during gestation.' Third International Symposium on
        Alcohol and Aldehyde Metabolizing Systems, p. 17 (abstract).

1190.   MENDELSON, R.A., and HUBER, A.M. (1980) 'The effect of duration
        of alcohol administration on the deposition of trace ele-
        ments in the fetal rat.' Advances in Experimental Medicine
        and Biology. Volume 132: Alcohol and Aldehyde Metabolizing
        Systems-IV. Ed. R.G. Thurman. New York: Plenum Press,
        pp. 295-304.

1191.   MENDELSON, R.A., and HUBER, A.M. (1980) 'The effect of ethanol
        consumption on trace elements in the fetal rat.' Currents
        in Alcoholism. Volume 7: Recent Advances in Research and
        Treatment. Ed. M. Galanter. New York: Grune and Stratton,
        pp. 39-48.

1192.   MENDELSSOHN, A. (1912) (In a discussion on alcoholism and de-
        generacy.) In: Bericht über den XIII. Internationalen
        Kongress gegen den Alkoholismus (The Hague), p. 212.

1193. MENENDEZ, C.E. (1980) 'Effects of alcohol on the male
      reproductive system.' In: Alcoholism: A Perspective.
      Ed. F.S. Messiha and G.S. Tyner. Westbury, New York: PJD
      Publications, pp. 69-77.

1194. MERIARI, A., GINTON, A., TAMAR, H., and TOVA, L.-R. (1973)
      'Effects of alcohol on mating behavior of the female rat.'
      Quarterly Journal of Studies on Alcohol, 34, 1095-1098.

1195. MERKATZ, I.R., MANN, L.I., LAUERSEN, N.H., and FUCHS, F. (1976)
      'Comparison of ritodrine and ethanol in premature labor.'
      Gynecological Investigation (Basel), 7 (Abstract #21).

1196. MESSIHA, F.S., and GIRGIS, S.M. (1978) 'Aldehyde dehydrogenase
      activity in the male rat reproductive tissues.' Proceedings
      of the Western Pharmacology Society, 21, 353-356.

1197. MESSIHA, F.S., LOX, C.D., and SPROAT, H.F. (1980) 'Effect of
      castration and oral contraceptives on hepatic ethanol and
      acetaldehyde metabolizing enzymes in the male rat.' Sub-
      stance Alcohol Action/Misuse, 1, 197-202.

1198. MESSIHA, F.S., TYNER, G.S., and GIRGIS, S.M. (1980) 'Property
      and specificity of aldehyde dehydrogenase in the rat
      testis.' In: Alcoholism: A Perspective. Ed. F.S. Mes-
      siha and G.S. Tyner. Westbury, New York: PJD Publications,
      pp. 467-477.

1199. MICELI, L.A., MARSH, E.J., and JARRETT, T.E. (1978) 'Fetal
      alcohol syndrome--physical and intellectual manifestations:
      Comparison of two cases.' Journal of the American Osteo-
      pathic Association, 78, 116-121.

1200. MICHAELIS, R., HAUG, S., MAJEWSKI, F., BIERICH, J.R., and DOP-
      FER, R. (1980) 'Obstetrische und postnatale Komplikationen
      bei Kindern mit einer Alkoholembryopathie.' ['Obstetrical
      and postnatal complications in infants with an alcohol em-
      bryopathy.'] Monatsschrift Kinderheilkunde, 128, 21-26.

1201. MIHAI, K. (1979) 'Embryopathia alcoholica. I. Anyai jellemzők.
      Klinikai tünetek.' ['Embryopathia alcoholica. Part I.
      Mother's characteristics and clinical symptoms.'] Alko-
      hologia (Budapest), 10, 214-218.

1202. MIHAI, K. (1980) 'Embryopathia alcoholica. II. Patogenezis.
      Összefügges a szindroma es a szerotonin anyagcsere között.'
      ['Embryopathia alcoholica. Part II. Pathogenesis. Cor-
      relation between syndrome and serotonin metabolism.'] Alko-
      hologia (Budapest), 11, 11-13.

1203. MILLER, J.C., and FRIEDHOFF, A.J. (1980) 'The effect of pre-
      natal exposure to ethanol or opiates on brain catecholamine
      activity.' Biogenic Amines Development 109-124.

1204. MILLER, R.K.   (1979)   'Drugs as teratogens: Three common syn-
       dromes.' Drug Therapy (Hospital), 4, 57-64.

1205. MIRONE, L. (1952) 'The effect of ethyl alcohol on growth,
       fecundity, and voluntary consumption of alcohol by mice.'
       Quarterly Journal of Studies on Alcohol, 13, 365-369.

1206. MIRONE, L. (1958) 'The effect of ethyl alcohol on growth and
       voluntary consumption of alcohol by successive generations
       of mice.' Quarterly Journal of Studies on Alcohol, 19,
       388-393.

1207. MODENESI, P. (1979) 'Localizzazione istochimica dell'alcool deidro-
       genasi durante l'invecchiamento del seme.' (Histochemical local-
       ization of ADH in aging sperm). Bollettino della Societa Itali-
       ana di Biologica Sperimentale, 55, 2395-2400.

1208. MØLLER, J., BRANDT, N.J., and TYGSTRUP, I. (1979) 'Hepatic
       dysfunction in patient with fetal alcohol syndrome.' Lan-
       cet (London), 1, 605-606.

1209. MOLNAR, J., and PAPP, G. (1973) 'Alkohol als möglicher schleim-
       fördernder Faktor im Samen.' ['Alcohol as a possible stimu-
       lant of mucus production in the semen.'] Andrologia (Ber-
       lin), 5, 105-106.

1210. MONJAN, A.A. and MANDELL, W. (1980) 'Fetal alcohol and immun-
       ity: Depression of mitogen-induced lymphocyte blasto-
       genesis.' Teratology, 21, 57A (abstract). (Also in Neuro-
       behavioral Toxicology, 2, 213-215.)

1211. MONTAGUE, D.K., JAMES, R.E., JR., DE-WOLFE, V.G., and MARTIN, L.M.
       (1979) 'Diagnostic evaluation, classification, and treat-
       ment of men with sexual dysfunction.' Urology, 14, 545-548.

1212. MOREL, B.A. (1857) Traite des degénérescences physiques, intel-
       lectuelles et morales de l'espèce humaine. [Stage of Phys-
       ical, Intellectual, and Moral Degeneration of the Human
       Species.] Paris.

1213. MOREL, B.A. (1860) Traite des maladies mentales. [Stage of
       Mental Maladies.] Paris.

1214. MOREL, B.A. (1867) L'heredité morbide progressive archives
       générales de médicine. [Progressively Morbid Heredity in
       the General Archives of Medicine.] Paris.

1215. MORIYAMA, I.S., ISHIBASHI, R., SHINTANI, M., and YAMAGUCHI, R.
       (1977) 'Studies on prolonged pregnancy: Comparison of
       methods for inducing prolonged pregnancy in rats.' Tera-
       tology, 16, 115.

1216. MØRLAND, J. (1980) 'Alkohol og fosterskader.' ['Alcohol and
       fetal damage.'] Tidsskrift for den norske Lægeforening,
       100, 299.

1217. MØRLAND, J.   (1980)   'Fosterskader fremkalt av alkohol.'   ['Fetal
       lesions due to alcohol.']   Tidsskrift for den norske Læge-
       forening, 100, 268-270.

1218. MORRA, M.   (1969)   'Ethanol and maternal stress on rat offspring
       behaviors.'   Journal of Genetic Psychology, 114, 77-83.

1219. MORRIS, C.   (1759)   A Collection of the Yearly Bills of Mortality
       from 1657 to 1758 Inclusive. To Which are Subjoined. . . .
       III. Observations on the Past Growth and Present State of
       the City of London. Reprinted from the edition printed at
       London in 1751. London: A. Millar.

1220. MORRISON, A.B., and MAYKUT, M.O.   (1979)   'Effets nocifs poten-
       tiels de l'ingestion d'alcool par la mère sur le développe-
       ment du foetus et séquelles chez le nouveau-né et l'enfant.'
       ['Potential adverse effects of maternal alcohol ingestion
       on the development of the fetus and their sequelae in the
       newborn and the child.']   L'Union médicale du Canada, 108,
       443-445. (Also in Canadian Medical Association Journal
       (Toronto), 120, 826-828.)

1221. MORRISSEY, E.R., and SCHUCKIT, M.A.   (1978)   'Stressful life
       events and alcohol problems among women seen at a detoxifi-
       cation center.'   Journal of Studies on Alcohol, 39, 1559.

1222. MORRISSEY, R.E.   (1980)   'Potential invertebrate model for as-
       sessing the effects of alcohol on nerve growth and synapse
       formation.'   Teratology, 21, 57A-58A (abstract).

1223. MORRISSEY, R.E., and MOTTET, N.K.   (1980)   'Neural tube defects
       and brain anomalies: A review of selected teratogens and
       their possible modes of action.'   Neurotoxicology, 2, 125-
       162.

1224. MOSKOVIC, S.   (1975)   'Uticaj hronicnog trovanja alkoholom na
       ovarijunsku disfunkciju.'   ['Effect of chronic alcohol in-
       toxication on ovarian dysfunction.']   Srpski Arhiv za celo-
       kupno Lekarstvo (Belgrad), 103, 751-758.

1225. MOSKOVIC, S.   (1977)   Hronicni alkoholizam i povecan broj spon-
       tanih pobacaja.'   ['Chronic alcoholism and increase in spon-
       taneous abortions.']   Srpski Arhiv za celokupno Lekarstvo
       (Belgrad), 105, 157-162.

1226. MOWAT, N.A., EDWARDS, C.R., and FISHER, R.   (1976)   'Hypothal-
       amic-pituitary-gonadal function in men with cirrhosis of the
       liver.'   Gut (London), 17, 345-350.

1227. MULVIHILL, J.J., KLIMAS, J.T., STOKES, D.C., and RISEMBERG, H.M.
       (1976)   'Fetal alcohol syndrome: Seven new cases.'   Amer-
       ican Journal of Obstetrics and Gynecology, 125, 937-941.

1228. MULVIHILL, J.J., and YEAGER, A.M.   (1976)   'Fetal alcohol syn-
       drome.'   Teratology, 13, 345-348.

1229. MUNJACK, D.J.   (1979)   'Sex and drugs.'   Clinical Toxicology, 15,
           75-89.

1230. MURPHREE, H.B.   (1968)   'Addiction and sexual behavior.'   In:
           Sexual Behavior and the Law.   Ed. R. Slovenko.   Springfield,
           Illinois: C.C. Thomas, pp. 591-606.

1231. MURPHY, W.D., COLEMAN, E., HOON, E., and SCOTT, C.   (1980)
           'Sexual dysfunction and treatment in alcoholic women.'
           Sexuality and Disability, 3, 240-255.

1232. MURRAY-LYON, I.M., BARRISON, I.G., WRIGHT, J.T., MORRIS, N.,
           and GORDON, M.   (1980)   'Alcohol abuse in pregnancy: A
           problem in London.'   [Letter.]   Lancet (London), 2, 1382.

1233. NAESS, K. (1977) 'Impotens fremkalt av medikamenter.' ['Im-
       potence caused by drugs.'] Tidsskrift for den Norske Laege-
       forening, 97, 468-469.

1234. NAKAMURA, H. (1975) 'Analysis of limb anomalies induced in
       vitro by vitamin A (retinol) in mice.' Teratology, 12,
       61-70.

1235. NAKAMURA, K., and SUZUKI, A. (1967) 'Expériences des malfor-
       mations congénitales de l'encéphale provoquées par inter-
       vention de certains agents (Étude sur le foetus du Rat de
       Wistar).' ['Experiments concerning congenital malformations
       of the encephalon induced by the intervention of certain
       agents: Studies on the Wistar Rat fetus.'] Archives
       d'Anatomie et de Cytologie Pathologiques (Paris), 15, 116-
       121.

1236. NATIONAL CLEARINGHOUSE FOR ALCOHOL INFORMATION. (1977) 'Nation-
       al awareness of fetal syndrome sought.' By E.P. Noble.
       NIAAA Information and Feature Service, September 8, p. 1.

1237. NATIONAL CLEARINGHOUSE FOR ALCOHOL INFORMATION. (1978) 'Social
       drinking affects behavior of newborn.' NIAAA Information
       and Feature Service, March 3, p. 3.

1238. NATIONAL CLEARINGHOUSE FOR ALCOHOL INFORMATION. (1978) 'Pamph-
       let warns on drinking in pregnancy.' NIAAA Information and
       Feature Service, April 3, p. 1.

1239. NATIONAL CLEARINGHOUSE FOR ALCOHOL INFORMATION. (1978) 'Defects
       frequent in babies of heavy drinkers.' NIAAA Information
       and Feature Service, May 31, p. 5.

1240. NATIONAL CLEARINGHOUSE FOR ALCOHOL INFORMATION. (1980) 'Fetal
       alcohol effects linked to moderate drinking levels.' By
       Sharon W. Rohner. NIAAA Information and Feature Service,
       June 9, p. 4.

1241. NATIONAL CLEARINGHOUSE FOR ALCOHOL INFORMATION. (1980) 'In-
         dians are focus of FAE screening project.' NIAAA Infor-
         mation and Feature Service, June 9, p. 5.

1242. NATIONAL CLEARINGHOUSE FOR ALCOHOL INFORMATION. (1980) 'Nation-
         wide FAE education effort underway.' NIAAA Information and
         Feature Service, June 9, p. 5.

1243. NATIONAL CLEARINGHOUSE FOR ALCOHOL INFORMATION. (1980) 'States
         offer varied FAE activities.' NIAAA Information and Fea-
         ture Service, June 9, p. 4.

1244. NATIONAL CLEARINGHOUSE FOR ALCOHOL INFORMATION. (1980) 'States
         continue to develop FAE awareness programs.' NIAAA Infor-
         mation and Feature Service, July 18, p. 5.

1245. NATIONAL COUNCIL ON ALCOHOLISM. (1978) You, Your Baby and
         Drinking. [Pamphlet.]

1246. NATIONAL FOUNDATION/MARCH OF DIMES. (1977) 'When you drink
         your unborn baby does, too!' [Brochure.] Box 2000, White
         Plains, New York 10602.

1247. NATIONAL INSTITUTE OF CHILD HEALTH AND HUMAN DEVELOPMENT. (1979)
         'Fetal-alcohol syndrome.' Pediatric Annals, 8, 119-120.

1248. NATIONAL INSTITUTE ON ALCOHOL ABUSE AND ALCOHOLISM. (1974)
         Second Special Report to the U.S. Congress on Alcohol and
         Health, from the Secretary of Health, Education, and Wel-
         fare. DHEW Publication No. (ADM) 74-124. U.S. Government
         Printing Office, Washington, D.C.

1249. NATIONAL INSTITUTE ON ALCOHOL ABUSE AND ALCOHOLISM. (1977)
         'Critical review of the fetal alcohol syndrome.' Rockville,
         Maryland: Alcohol, Drug Abuse, and Mental Health Adminis-
         tration, pp. 1-58.

1250. NATIONAL ORGANIZATION OF DISTILLED SPIRITS INDUSTRY. (1978)
         'Warning label opposed: Ineffective, not needed.' Discus
         News Letter, March, No. 373.

1251. NATIONAL ORGANIZATION OF DISTILLED SPIRITS INDUSTRY. (1978)
         'ACA: Perspective on F.A.S., warning labels.' Discus News
         Letter, April, No. 374.

1252. NATIONAL SWEDISH BOARD OF HEALTH AND WELFARE (SOCIALSTYRELSEN).
         (1980) 'Missbruk under graviditet.' ['Abuse in pregnancy.']
         Stockholm, pp. 1-39.

1253. NAZARYAN, S.S. (1976) 'O nekotirykh disgarmoniyakh seksual'noi
         zhizni u bol'nykh alkogolizmom.' ['Some of the disorders in
         the sex life of alcoholics.'] Zhurnal Eksperimental'noi i
         Klinicheskoi Meditsiny (Erevan), 16, 88-91.

1254. NEAL, R. (1977) 'Fetal alcohol syndrome.' NBC Nightly News. May 31.

1255. NEIDENGARD, L., CARTER, T.E., and SMITH, D.W. (1978) 'Klippel-Feil malformation complex in fetal alcohol syndrome.' American Journal of Diseases of Children, 132, 929-930.

1256. NELSON, B.J. (1981) 'How alcohol affects sexually: Scientists investigate the paradox.' Sexual Medicine Today, May, pp. 6-7, 10, 30.

1257. NELSON, B.K., BRIGHTWELL, W.S., SETZER, J.V., HORNUNG, R.W., and O'DONOHUE, T.L. (1981) 'Interactive effects of ethanol on the behavioral teratogenic effects of the industrial solvent 2-ethoxy-ethanol in rats.' Teratology, 24, 57A (abstract).

1258. NELSON, V.S., PALUSZNY, M.J., RHODES, W.C., and STREISSGUTH, A.P. (1978) 'Special needs of the F.A.S. child and family.' Paper presented at the Fetal Alcohol Syndrome Symposium, Ann Arbor, Michigan.

1259. NESHKOV, N.S. (1969) 'Sostoyaniye spermatogeneza i polovoi funktsii u zloupotreblyayushchikh alkogolem.' ['State of spermatogenesis and sexual function in alcoholic abusers.'] Vrachebnoe Delo (Kiev), 2, 130-131.

1260. NESTERICK, C.A. (1980) 'The role of the tetrahydroisoquinoline, salsolinol, in the mechanism of ethanol teratogenicity.' Ph.D. dissertation, Ohio State University, Dissertation Abstracts International, 40, 5227B.

1261. NETZLOFF, M.L., STREIFF, R.R., FRIAS, J.L., and RENNERT, O.M. (1979) 'Folate anatagonism following teratogenic exposure to diphenylhydantoin.' Teratology, 19, 45-50.

1262. NEUGUT, R.H. (1980) 'A critical review of the literature on the fetal alcohol syndrome in humans.' In: An Assessment of Statistics on Alcohol-Related Problems. Ed. E. Joseph-son. Prepared for the Distilled Spirits Council of the United States. (Paged by sections.) [Washington, D.C.], pp. I-1-I-57.

1263. NEUHÄUSER, G. (1974) 'Missbildungen durch Alkohol.' ['Defects from alcohol.'] Hippokrates (Stuttgart), 45, 496-497.

1264. NEWMAN, N.M., and CORREY, J.F. (1980) 'Effects of alcohol in pregnancy.' Medical Journal of Australia, 2, 5-10.

1265. NEWMAN, S.L., FLANNERY, D.B., and CAPLAN, D.B. (1979) 'Simul-taneous occurrence of extrahepatic biliary atresia and fetal alcohol syndrome.' American Journal of Diseases of Chil-dren, 133, 101.

1266. NEWSWEEK. (1973) 'Eight babies of alcoholic mothers have serious malformations.' July 16, p. 93.

1267. NEWSWEEK. (1973) 'Martinis and motherhood.' July 16.

1268. NEW YORK STATE DIVISION OF ALCOHOLISM AND ALCOHOL ABUSE. (1981)
       'Fetal alcohol syndrome: Teaching packet.' Albany,
       New York: New York State Division of Alcoholism and Alco-
       hol Abuse.

1269. NEW YORK STATE TASK FORCE ON FETAL ALCOHOL SYNDROME/ALCOHOL
       RELATED BIRTH DEFECTS. (1979) Fetal Alcohol Syndrome:
       Task Force Report to the Governor. Albany, New York:
       New York State Division of Alcoholism and Alcohol Abuse.

1270. NICE, L.B. (1912) 'Comparative studies on the effects of alco-
       hol, nicotine, tobacco smoke and caffeine on white mice.'
       Journal of Experimental Zoology, 12, 133-152.

1271. NICE, L.B. (1917) 'Further observations on the effects of
       alcohol on white mice.' American Naturalist, 51, 596-607.

1272. NICHOLS, M.M. (1967) 'Acute alcohol withdrawal syndrome in a
       newborn.' American Journal of Diseases of Children, 113,
       714-715.

1273. NICLOUX, M. (1899) 'Sur le passage de l'alcool ingeré de la
       mère au foetus, en particulier chez la femme.' ['Passage
       of alcohol, ingested by the mother, to the fetus, particu-
       larly in females.'] Comptes Rendus des Séances de la
       Société de Biologie et de Ses Filiales (Paris), 51, 980-
       982.

1274. NICLOUX, M. (1900) 'Passage de l'alcool ingeré de la mère au
       foetus et passage de l'alcool ingeré dans le lait, en par-
       ticulier chez la femme.' ['Passage of alcohol, ingested by
       the mother, to the fetus, and passage of alcohol ingested
       in milk, particularly in females.'] Obstétrique, 5, 97-132.

1275. NIEBYL, J.R., and JOHNSON, J.W.C. (1980) 'Inhibition of preterm
       labor.' Clinical Obstetrics and Gynecology, 23, 115-126.

1276. NIIMI, Y. (1973) 'Studies on effects of alcohol on fetus.'
       [In Japanese.] Sanfujinka no Shinpo [Advances in Obstetrics
       and Gynecology], 25, 55-78.

1277. NIIMI, Y. (1975) 'Statistical observations on the course of
       labor in the women who consume alcohol.' [In Japanese.]
       Sanka to Fujinka [Obstetrics and Gynecology], 42, 1249-1253.

1278. NISHIMURA, H., and TANIMURA, T. (1976) Clinical Aspects of the
       Teratology of Drugs. New York: American Elsevier Pub-
       lishing Company.

1279. NISWANDER, K.R. (1977) 'Obstetric factors related to prematur-
       ity.' In: The Epidemiology of Prematurity. Ed. D.M. Reed
       and F.J. Stanley. Baltimore: Urban and Schwarzenberg,
       pp. 249-264.

1280. NITOWSKY, H.M.   (1980)   'Teratogenic effects of ethanol in human beings.'   Neurobehavioral Toxicology, 2, 151-155.

1281. NITOWSKY, H.M.   (1980)   'The fetal alcohol syndrome--an overview.'   Teratology, 21, 59a (abstract).

1282. NIWELINSK, J.   (1980)   'Alkoholizm a vozwoj płodowy.'   ['Alcoholism and development of the fetus.']   Polska Problemy Alkoholizmu (Warsaw), 27, 5.

1283. NOBLE, E.P., ed.   (1978)   'Fetal alcohol syndrome and other effects on offspring.'   Alcohol and Health: Third Special Report to the U.S. Congress on Alcohol and Health.   Washington, D.C.:   U.S. Government Printing Office, NIAAA, pp. 171-193.

1284. NOBLE, E.P.   (1981)   'Summary and final comments [on FAS Workshop].'   Neurobehavioral Toxicology and Teratology, 3, 247-248.

1285. NOONAN, J.A.   (1976)   'Congenital heart disease in the fetal alcohol syndrome.'   American Journal of Cardiology, 37, 160.

1286. NOONAN, J.A.   (1978)   'Association of congenital heart disease with syndromes or other defects.'   Pediatric Clinics of North America, 25, 797-816.

1287. NORA, A.H., NORA, J.J., and BLU, J.   (1977)   'Limb-reduction anomalies in infants born to disulfiram-treated alcoholic mothers.'   [Letter.]   Lancet (London), 2, 664.

1288. NORA, J.J., NORA, A.H., BLU, J., INGRAM, J., FOUNTAIN, A., PETERSON, M., LORTSCHER, R.H., and KIMBERLING, W.J.   (1978)   'Exogenous progestogen and estrogen implicated in birth defects.'   Journal of the American Medical Association, 240, 837-843.

1289. NORDIN, R., and CAMPBELL, R.   (1980)   'Preliminary observations of working with childbearing clients who are involved with alcohol abuse or alcohol recovery.'   Paper presented at the National Council on Alcohol Conference, Seattle, Washington.

1290. NORONHA, A.B., and DRUSE-MANTEUFFEL, M.J.   (1980)   'Chronic maternal ethanol consumption through the second trimester of gestation: Synaptic plasma membrane proteins and glycoproteins in offspring.'   Society for Neuroscience, Cincinnati, Ohio (November 9-14).

1291. NORPPA, H., SORSA, M., and VAINIO, H.   (1980)   'Chromosomal aberrations in bone marrow of chinese hamsters exposed to styrene and ethanol.'   Toxicology Letters, 5, 241-244.

1292. NOSAL, G. (1976) 'Drogues et maternité: Un dilemme pour la
          femme? Données actuelles et perspectives.' ['Drugs and
          maternity: A dilemma for women? Current data and perspec-
          tives.'] <u>Toxicomanies</u> (Quebec), <u>9</u>, 175-225.

O

1293. OAKLEY, G.P., JR. (1980) 'Causal interference in teratology.' Progress in Clinical and Biological Research. Volume 36: Drug and Chemical Risks to the Newborn--Proceedings of a Symposium. Ed. R.H. Schwarz and S.J. Yaffe. New York: Alan R. Liss, pp. 33-40.

1294. OBE, G., and BEEK, B. (1979) 'Mutagenic activity of aldehydes.' Drug and Alcohol Dependence (Lausanne), 4, 91-94.

1295. OBE, G., and HERHA, J. (1975) 'Chromosomal damage in chronic alcohol users.' Humangenetik (Berlin), 29, 191-200.

1296. OBE, G., and MAJEWSKI, F. (1978) 'No elevation of exchange type--aberrations in the lymphocytes of children with alcohol embryopathy.' Humangenetik (Berlin), 43, 31-36.

1297. OBE, G., NATARAJAN, A.T., MEYERS, M., and HERTOG, A.D. (1979) 'Induction of chromosomal aberrations in peripheral lymphocytes of human blood in vitro, and of SCE's in bone-marrow cells of mice in vivo by ethanol and its metabolite acetaldehyde.' Mutation Research (Amsterdam), 68, 291-294.

1298. OBE, G., and RISTOW, H. (1977) 'Acetaldehyde but not ethanol induces sister chromatid exchanges in Chinese hamster cells in vitro.' Mutation Research (Amsterdam), 56, 211-214.

1299. OBE, G., and RISTOW, H. (1979) 'Mutagenic, carcinogenic, and teratogenic effects of alcohol.' Mutation Research (Amsterdam), 65, 229-259.

1300. OBSTETRICAL AND GYNECOLOGICAL NEWS. (1976) 'Infant of excessive drinker prone to anomalies.' February 1, p. 44.

1301. OGATA, S. (1919) 'Preliminary report of studies on the influence of alcohol and nicotine in the ovary.' Journal of Medical Research, 40, 123-127.

1302. O'GORMAN, P. (1980) 'Perspectives on prevention.' Paper pre-
       sented at the 20th Annual Meeting of the Teratology Society,
       Portsmouth, New Hampshire (June 8-12).

1303. ØISUND, J.F., FJORDEN, A.-E., and MØRLAND, J. (1978) 'Is mod-
       erate ethanol consumption teratogenic in the rat?' Acta
       Pharmacologica et Toxicologia (Copenhagen), 43, 145-155.

1304. OKADA, D.M. (1977) 'The fetal alcohol syndrome.' The Inter-
       national Medical Symposium on Alcohol and Drug Dependence
       (ICAA Symposium in Japan), p. 150 (abstract).

1305. OKADA, R. (1978) 'Fetal alcohol syndrome.' [In Japanese.]
       Nippon Rinsho, Supplement, pp. 1494-1495.

1306. OLEGÅRD, R. (1978) 'Sambandet mellan alkohol och fosterskador.'
       [The relationship between alcohol and embryopathy.'] Al-
       kohol och Narkotika, 72, 10-12.

1307. OLEGÅRD, R. (1980) 'Clinical studies of FAS in Sweden.' Paper
       presented at the Fetal Alcohol Syndrome Workshop, Seattle,
       Washington (May 2-4).

1308. OLEGÅRD, R. (1980) 'Effects of alcohol abuse during pregnancy:
       A prospective study in Sweden.' Paper presented at the
       Fetal Alcohol Syndrome Workshop, Seattle, Washington
       (May 2-4).

1309. OLEGÅRD, R., SABEL, K.-G., ARONSSON, M., SANDIN, B., JOHANSSON,
       P.R., CARLSSON, C., KYLLERMAN, M., IVERSEN, K., and HRBEK,
       A. (1979) 'Effects on the child of alcohol abuse during
       pregnancy: Retrospective and prospective studies.' Acta
       Paediatrica Scandinavica, Supplement No. 275, 112-121.

1310. OLEGÅRD, R., SABEL, K.-G., SANDIN, B., ARONSSON, M., and KYLLER-
       MAN, M. (1980) 'Outcome of children to alcoholic mothers
       related to social conditions during upbringing.' Pediatric
       Research, 14, 1415 (abstract).

1311. OLIVO, J., GORDON, G.G., RAFII, I., and SOUTHERN, A.L. (1975)
       'Estrogen metabolism in hyperthyroidism and in cirrhosis
       of the liver.' Steroids, 26, 47-56.

1312. OLOW, J. (1923) 'Über das Übergang des Ethylalkohols in die
       Milch abstillender Frauen.' ['On the passage of ethyl
       alcohol in the milk of nursing women.'] Biochemische
       Zeitung, 134, 553-558.

1313. OLOW, J. (1923) Über das Übergehen des Äthylalkohols von der
       Mutter zur Frucht.' ['On the passage of ethyl alcohol from
       the mother to the fetus.'] Biochemische Zeitschrift, 134,
       407-414.

1314. OMENN, G.J. (1975) 'Alcoholism: A pharmacogenetic disorder.'
       Modern Problems in Pharmacopsychiatry (Berlin), 10, 12-22.

1315.   OPINION RESEARCH CORPORATION.   (1979)   'General public caravan
           survey #71053.' Unpublished tables completed under contract
           to the Bureau of Alcohol, Tobacco, and Firearms (July).

1316.   OSBORNE, G.L.   (1978)   'An evaluation of the role of early ex-
           perience in determining behavioral effects of prenatal
           ethanol exposure.' Ph.D. dissertation, Vanderbilt Univer-
           sity. Dissertation Abstracts International (B), 39, 5635
           (abstract).

1317.   OSBORNE, G.L., CAUL, W.F., and FERNANDEZ, K.   (1980)   'Behav-
           ioral effects of prenatal ethanol exposure and differential
           early experience in rats.' Pharmacology, Biochemistry, and
           Behavior, 12, 393-401.

1318.   O'SHEA, K.S., and KAUFMAN, M.H.   (1979)   'The teratogenic effect
           of acetaldehyde: Implications for the study of the fetal
           alcohol syndrome.' Journal of Anatomy (London), 128, 65-76.

1319.   O'SHEA, K.S., and KAUFMAN, M.H.   (1981)   'Effect of acetaldehyde
           on the neuroepithelium of early mouse embryos.' Journal of
           Anatomy (London), 132, 107-118.

1320.   OTT, A., HAYES, J., and POLIN, J.   (1976)   'Severe lactic acid-
           osis associated with intravenous alcohol for premature
           labor.' Obstetrics and Gynecology, 48, 362-364.

1321.   OUELLETTE, E.M.   (1979)   'Alcohol in pregnancy and its effects
           on offspring.' In: Fermented Food Beverages in Nutrition.
           Ed. C.F. Gastineau, W.J. Darby, and T.B. Turner. New York:
           Academic Press, pp. 439-454.

1322.   OUELLETTE, E.M., and ROSETT, H.L.   (1976)   'A pilot prospective
           study of the fetal alcohol syndrome at the Boston City
           Hospital. Part II: The infants.' Annals of the New York
           Academy of Sciences, 273, 123-129.

1323.   OUELLETTE, E.M., and ROSETT, H.L.   (1977)   'Study of the fetal
           alcohol syndrome at the Boston City Hospital.' Paper pre-
           sented at the NIAAA Fetal Alcohol Syndrome Workshop,
           San Diego, California.

1324.   OuELLETTE, E.M., and ROSETT, H.L.   (1977)   'The effect of
           maternal alcohol ingestion during pregnancy on offspring.'
           In: Nutritional Impacts on Women. Ed. K.S. Moshissi and
           T.N. Evans.   , Maryland: Harper and Row, pp. ?

1325.   OUELLETTE, E.M., ROSETT, H.L., ROSMAN, N.P., and WEINER, L.
           (1977)   'Adverse effects on offspring of maternal alcohol
           abuse during pregnancy.' New England Journal of Medicine,
           297, 528-530.

1326.   OVIZE, H.   (1900)   'Alcoolisme et depopulation.' ['Alcoholism
           and depopulation.'] Thèse, Lyons.

P

1327. PACE, D.M., and FROST, B.L. (1948) 'The effects of ethyl alcohol on growth and respiration in Pelomyxa carolinensis and upon conjugation in Paramecium caudatum.' Anatomical Record, 101, 730.

1328. PACHE, H.D. (1976) 'Alkohol-Embryopathie.' ['Alcohol embryopathy.'] Münchener Medizinische Wochenschrift, Supplement (Munich), 118, 7-8.

1329. PALMER, R.H., OUELLETTE, E.M., WARNER, L., and LEICHTMAN, S.R. (1974) 'Congenital malformations in offspring of a chronic alcoholic mother.' Pediatrics, 53, 490-494.

1330. PALMISANO, P.A., SNEED, R.C., and CASSADY, G. (1969) 'Untaxed whiskey and fetal lead exposure.' Journal of Pediatrics, 75, 869-872.

1331. PAPARA-NICHOLSON, D., and TELFORD, I.R. (1957) 'Effects of alcohol on reproduction and fetal development in the guinea pig.' Anatomical Record, 127, 438-439.

1332. PARKER, J.A. (1980) 'Influence of zinc on the teratogenic and mutagenic potential of ethanol in mice.' Ph.D. dissertation, University of California, Davis. Dissertation Abstracts International, 41, 817-B.

1333. PASHCHENKOV, S.Z. (1980) 'Ob alkogolnii embryopathiia.' ['Alcoholic embryopathies.'] Pediatriia, 12, 47-49.

1334. PASHCHENKOV, S.Z. (1981) 'Alkogolnii embryopathia.' ['Alcoholic embryopathies.'] Akusherstvo Ginekologiia (Moscow), 1, 35-36.

1335. PASSE, L.M. (1980) 'Commonly asked questions about alcohol and pregnancy.' Street Pharmacologist, 3, 3-4.

1336. PATEL, N.B., and MAC NAUGHTON, M.C.   (1969)   'Premature labor--
       a new technique; the use of intravenous alcohol infusion
       in the prevention of premature labour.'   Nursing Times
       (London), 65, 650-652.

1337. PATRY, E., and FERRIER, A.   (1934)   'Action de l'alcool ethylique
       sur le developpement de l'embryon de poulet.'   ['Action of
       ethyl alcohol on the development of the chicken embryo.']
       Comptes Rendus des Séances de la Société de Biologie et de
       Ses Filiales (Paris), 116, 928.

1338. PAULUS, W.D.   (1976)   'Effect of maternal ethanol inhalation
       during pregnancy in the craniofacial development in the
       A/J mouse.'   M.A. Thesis, Case Western Reserve University.

1339. PAWLAK, V.   (1978)   'Fetal alcohol syndrome.'   Street Pharma-
       cologist, 1.

1340. PAWLAK, V.   (1980)   'Fetal alcohol syndrome: New developments.'
       Street Pharmacologist, 3, 1-2.

1341. PAWLAK-FRAZIER, P., and PAWLAK-FRAZIER, D.   (1978)   'Cause and
       defect: Foetal alcohol syndrome.'   All Faith's World Alco-
       hol Project Journal, 1, 25-29.

1342. PEARL, R.   (1916)   'On the effect of continued administration of
       certain poisons to the domestic fowl, with special refer-
       ence to the progeny.'   Proceedings of the American Philo-
       sophical Society, 4, 243-258.

1343. PEARL, R.   (1916)   'Some effects of the continued administration
       of alcohol to the domestic fowl, with special reference
       to the progeny.'   Proceedings of the National Academy of
       Sciences of the United States of America, 2, 380-384.

1344. PEARL, R.   (1916)   'The effect of parental alcoholism (and cer-
       tain other drug intoxications) upon the progeny in the
       domestic fowl.'   Proceedings of the National Academy of
       Sciences of the United States of America, 2, 675-683.

1345. PEARL, R.   (1917)   'The effect of parental alcoholism and cer-
       tain other drug intoxications upon the progeny.'   Journal
       of Experimental Zoology, 22, 24.

1346. PEARL, R.   (1917)   'The experimental modification of germ cells.
       I. General plan of experiments with ethyl alcohol and cer-
       tain related substances.'   Journal of Experimental Zoology,
       22, 125-164.

1347. PEARL, R.   (1917)   'The experimental modification of germ cells.
       II. The effect upon the domestic fowl of the daily inhala-
       tion of ethyl alcohol and certain related substances.'
       Journal of Experimental Zoology, 22, 165-186.

1348. PEARL, R. (1917) 'The experimental modification of germ cells. III. The effect of parental alcoholism, and certain other drug intoxications, upon the progeny.' Journal of Experimental Zoology, 22, 241-310.

1349. PEARSON, K. (1910-1911) 'Alcohol and offspring.' British Journal of Inebriety, 8, 53-66.

1350. PEARSON, K. (1911) 'Alcohol and degeneracy.' British Medical Journal (London), 1, 332.

1351. PEARSON, K. (1911) Letter concerning Edinburgh data used by Elderton and Pearson. British Medical Journal (London), 1, 333-336.

1352. PEARSON, K., and ELDERTON, E.M. (1910) 'A second study of the influence of parental alcoholism on the physique and ability of the offspring. A reply to medical critics of the first memoir.' Eugenics Laboratory Memoirs, 13, 35.

1353. PEDEN, V.H., SAMMON, T.J., and DOWNEY, D.A. (1973) 'Intravenously induced infantile intoxication with ethanol.' Journal of Pediatrics, 83, 490-493.

1354. PEIFFER, J., MAJEWSKI, F., FISCHBACH, H., BIERICH, J.R., and VOLK, B. (1979) 'Alcohol embryo- and fetopathy: Neuropathology of three children and three fetuses.' Journal of Neurological Science (Amsterdam), 41, 125-137.

1355. PELKONEN, O., JOUPPILA, P., and KAERKI, N.T. (1973) 'Attempts to induce drug metabolism in human fetal liver and placenta by the administration of phenobarbital to mothers.' Arhives Internationales de Pharmacodynamie et de Thérapie, 202, 288-297.

1356. PELOSI, M., LANGER, A., APUZZIO, J., KAMINETZKY, H., and FRICCHIONE, D. (1980) 'Drinking and pregnancy.' Journal of the Medical Society of New Jersey, 77, 101-102.

1357. PENNINGTON, S.N., SMITH, C.P., JR., and STRIDER, J.B., JR. (1980) 'Alterations in maternal and fetal prostaglandin dehydrogenase as a result of maternal ethanol consumption.' Alcoholism: Clinical and Experimental Research, 4, 225 (abstract).

1358. PENNINGTON, S.N., SMITH, C.P., JR., and STRIDER, J.B., JR. (1980) 'The effect of ethanol on the metabolism of prostaglandins and selected compounds.' In: Advances in Experimental Medicine and Biology. Volume 132: Alcohol and Aldehyde Metabolizing Systems-IV. New York: Plenum Press, pp. 527-532.

1359. PENTIKAMEN, P.J., PENTIKAMEN, L.A., and AZARNOTT, D.L. (1975) 'Plasma levels and excretion of estrogens in urine in chronic liver disease.' Gastroenterology, 69, 20-27.

1360. PERLIN, M.J., and SIMON, K.J.   (1979) 'The epidemiology of
       drug use during pregnancy.' International Journal of the
       Addictions, 14, 355-364.

1361. PERSIANINOV, L.S., KIRIUSHCHENKOV, A.P., and SKOSYREVA, A.M.
       (1974) 'Cultivation of rat embryos in vitro by New's
       method in pharmacology.' [In Russian.] Arkhiv Anatomii
       Gistologii Embriologii, 66, 93-97.

1362. PERSKY, H., O'BRIEN, C.P., FINE, E. et al. (1977) 'The effect
       of alcohol and smoking on testosterone function and aggres-
       sion in chronic alcoholics.' American Journal of Psychia-
       try, 134, 621-625.

1363. PESCE, V.S. (1980) 'L'uso della droga ed i suoi riflesse
       sull'apparato genitale femminile.' ['The use of drugs and
       its effects on the female genital system.' Minerva Medica
       (Torino), 71, 2381-2388.

1364. PETERSEN, D.R., PANTER, S.S., and COLLINS, A.C. (1977) 'Eth-
       anol and acetaldehyde metabolism in the pregnant mouse.'
       Drug and Alcohol Dependence, 2, 409-420.

1365. PETERSON, K.L., and SEEGMILLER, R.E. (1981) 'Fetotoxicity fol-
       lowing chronic prenatal exposure of mice to ethanol and
       tobacco smoke.' Teratology, 23, 56A (abstract).

1366. PFEIFER, W.D., MAC KINNON, J.R., and SEISER, R.L. (1977) 'Ad-
       verse effects of paternal alcohol consumption on offspring
       in the rat.' Bulletin of the Psychonomic Society, 10, 246.

1367. PHILLIPS, D.S., and STAINBROOK, G.L. (1976) 'Effects of early
       alcohol exposure upon adult learning ability and taste
       preferences.' Physiological Psychology, 4, 473-475.

1368. PHILLIPS, D.S., and STAINBROOK, G.L. (1978) 'Fecundity, natal-
       ity, and weight as a function of prenatal alcohol consump-
       tion and age of the mother.' Physiological Psychology, 6,
       75-77.

1369. PHIPPS, B.S. (1981) 'The effects of in utero ethanol exposure
       on the development of CA$_1$ pyramidal neurons of the hippo-
       campus.' Ph.D. Dissertation, Tufts University.

1370. PICK, J.R., and ELLIS, F.W. (1980) 'The fetal alcohol syndrome
       in beagles as affected by ethanol dose variations.' Tera-
       tology, 21, 61A (abstract).

1371. PICK, J.R., ELLIS, F.W., and DIEHL, W.J. (1978) 'Ethanol ex-
       posure during organogenesis in the Beagle model of the
       fetal alcohol syndrome.' Pharmacologist, 20, 194 (ab-
       stract).

1372. PICK, J.R., ELLIS, F.W., and SAWYER, M. (1977) 'The beagle as
       an animal model resembling the human fetal alcohol syn-
       drome.' Proceedings of the American Association of Labora-
       tory Animal Science Publications, 77-3 (Abstract #59).

1373. PICTET, A. (1924) 'Resultants negatifs d'experiences d'alcool-
       isme sur les cobayes. Sur l'appaution de cobayes anor maux
       dans des lignées non-alcooliques.' ['Absence of effects
       of exposure to alcohol on guinea pigs. On the birth of
       abnormal guinea pigs in the non-alcoholic luni.'] Comptes
       Rendus de la Société Physique et d'histoire Naturelle de
       Genève, 41, 29-33.

1374. PIEROG, S., CHANDAVASU, O., and WEXLER, I. (1977) 'Withdrawal
       symptoms in infants with the fetal alcohol syndrome.'
       Journal of Pediatrics, 90, 630-633.

1375. PIEROG, S., CHANDAVASU, O., and WEXLER, I. (1979) 'The fetal
       alcohol syndrome: Some maternal characteristics.' Inter-
       national Journal of Gynecology and Obstetrics, 16, 412-415.

1376. PIEROTTI, D. (1980) 'Fetal alcohol syndrome public awareness
       campaign.' Paper presented at the National Council on Alco-
       hol Conference, Seattle, Washington.

1377. PILSTROM, L., and KIESSLING, K.H. (1967) 'Effect of ethanol on
       the growth and on the liver and brain mitochondrial func-
       tions of the offspring of rats.' Acta Pharmacologica et
       Toxicologica (Copenhagen), 25, 225-232.

1378. PINHAS, V. (1978) 'Sex guilt and sexual control in the woman
       alcoholic in early sobriety.' Unpublished doctoral disser-
       tation, Department of Health Education, New York University.

1379. PINHAS, V. (1979) 'An investigation to compare the degree to
       which alcoholic and non-alcoholic women report sex guilt
       and sexual control.' Paper presented at the National Alco-
       holism Forum of the National Council on Alcoholism, Wash-
       ington, D.C. (April).

1380. PIZZARELLO, D.J., and FORD, R.V., JR. (1968) 'Effects of para-
       dimethylaminoazobenzene and the antioxidant N,N'-diphenyl-
       P-phenylene diamine in developing chicks.' Experientia,
       24, 621-622.

1381. PÓCSY, T., and BALASSA, É. (1978) 'Alkoholos embryopathia.'
       ['Alcoholic embryopathy.'] Orvosi Hetilap (Budapest), 119,
       209-211.

1382. PODOLSKY, E. (1963) 'The woman alcoholic and premenstrual ten-
       sion.' Journal of the American Medical Women's Association,
       18, 816-818.

1383. PODRATZ, K.C. (1978) 'Alcoholic ketoacidosis in pregnancy.'
       Obstetrics and Gynecology, 52 (Supplement), 54S-57S.

1384. POMERANCE, J.J., and YAFFE, S.J. (1973) 'Maternal medication
         and its effect on the fetus.' Current Problems in Ped-
         iatrics, 4, 3-60.

1385. PÖSÖ, H., and PÖSÖ, A.R. (1981) 'Inhibition of rat ovarian
         ornithine decarboxylase by ethanol in vivo and in vitro.'
         Biochimica et Biophysica Acta, 658, 291-298.

1386. POTTER, B.J., BELLING, G.B., MANO, M.T., and HETZEL, B.S. (1980)
         'Experimental production of growth retardation in the sheep
         fetus after exposure to alcohol.' Medical Journal of Aus-
         tralia, 2, 191-193.

1387. POTTER, J. (1979) 'Women and sex--It's enough to drive them to
         drink!' In: Women Who Drink: Alcoholic Experience and
         Psychotherapy. Ed. V. Burtle. Springfield, Illinois:
         Charles C. Thomas, pp. 49-?

1388. POTTS, W.A. (1909) 'The relationship of alcohol to feeble-
         mindedness.' British Journal of Inebriety, 6, 135-149.

1389. POWELL, B.J., VIAMONTES, J.A., and BROWN, C.S. (1974) 'Alcohol
         effects on the sexual potency of alcoholic and non-alcoholic
         males.' Alcoholism (Zagreb), 10, 78-80.

1390. POWELL, D.J. (1980) 'Sexual dysfunction and alcoholism.' Jour-
         nal of Sex Education and Therapy, 6, 40-46.

1391. PRASAD, D.R., KAUFMAN, R.H., and PRASAD, N. (1978) 'Effect of
         maternal alcohol exposure on fetal ovarian lactate dehydro-
         genase.' Obstetrics and Gynecology, 52, 318-320.

1392. PRATT, O.E. (1980) 'The fetal alcohol syndrome: Transport of
         nutrients and transfer of alcohol and acetaldehyde from
         mother to fetus.' In: Psychopharmacology of Alcohol.
         Ed. M. Sandler. New York: Raven Press, pp. 229-256.

1393. PREISIG, H., and AMADIAN, K. (1918-1919) 'Les alcooliques
         sont-ils dégénéres?' ['Alcoholics--are they degenerate?']
         Schweizerisches Archiv für Neurologie und Psychiatrie, 3,
         147-176.

1394. PRIMROSE, D.A. (1977) 'Fetal alcohol syndrome.' [Letter.]
         Developmental Medicine and Child Neurology (London), 19,
         695.

1395. PUIG, M., ARCE, A., DE JUANA, R., LEANDRO, S.V., and VILLA-
         ELÍZAGA, I. (1979) 'Síndrome de alcohol fetal.' ['Fetal
         alcohol syndrome.'] Revista de Medicina de la Universidad
         de Navarra, 23, 34-44.

1396. PUIG, M., ARCE, A., DE JUANA, R., LEANDRO, S.V., and VILLA-
         ELÍZAGA, I. (1981) 'Síndrome de alcohol fetal.' ['Fetal
         alcohol syndrome.'] Revista de Medicina de la Universidad
         de Navarra, 25, 198-208.

1397. PÜSCHEL, K., and SEIFERT, H.   (1979)   'Bedeutung des Alkohols in
        der Embryofetalperiode und beim Neugeborenen.'   ['Signifi-
        cance of alcohol on the embryo, fetus, and newborn.']   Zeit-
        schrift für Rechtsmedizin, 83, 69-76.

1398. PÜSPÖKY, G.   (1979)   'Embryopathia alcoholica.'   ['Alcoholic
        embryopathy.']   Orvosi Hetilap, 120, 775-777.

Q

1399. QAZI, Q.H., CHUA, A., MILMAN, D., and SOLISH, G. (1980) 'Outcome of pregnancy in heavy drinking women.' Alcoholism: Clinical and Experimental Research, 4, 226 (abstract).

1400. QAZI, Q.H., MADAHAR, C., MASAKAWA, A., and MC GANN, B. (1978) 'Chromosome abnormality in a patient with fetal alcohol syndrome.' Alcoholism: Clinical and Experimental Research, 2, 201 (abstract).

1401. QAZI, Q.H., MADAHAR, C., MASAKAWA, A., and MC GANN, B. (1979) 'Chromosome abnormality in a patient with fetal alcohol syndrome.' In: Currents in Alcoholism. Volume 5: Biomedical Issues and Clinical Effects of Alcoholism. Ed. M. Galanter. New York: Grune and Stratton, pp. 155-161.

1402. QAZI, Q.H., and MASAKAWA, A. (1976) 'Altered sex ratio in fetal alcohol syndrome.' Lancet (London), 1, 42.

1403. QAZI, Q.H., MASAKAWA, A., MC GANN, B., and WOODS, J. (1980) 'Dermatoglyphic abnormalities in the fetal alcohol syndrome.' Teratology, 21, 157-160.

1404. QAZI, Q.H., MASAKAWA, A., MILMAN, D.H., MC GANN, B., CHUA, A., and ALVI, S. (1978) 'Renal abnormalities in fetal alcohol syndrome.' Pediatric Research, 12, 517 (abstract).

1405. QAZI, Q., MASAKAWA, A., MILMAN, D.H., MC GANN, B., CHUA, A., and HALLER, J. (1979) 'Renal anomalies in fetal alcohol syndrome.' Pediatrics, 63, 886-889.

1406. QAZI, Q., MASAKAWA, A., MILMAN, D.H., MC GANN, B., and NEUMANN, S. (1977) 'Fetal alcohol syndrome.' The International Medical Symposium on Alcohol and Drug Dependence (ICAA Symposium in Japan), p. 129 (abstract).

R

1407. RACHAMIN, G., MAC DONALD, J.A., WAHID, S., CLAPP, J.J., KHANNA,
       J.M., and ISRAEL, Y. (1980) 'Modulation of alcohol dehy-
       drogenase and ethanol metabolism by sex hormones in the
       spontaneously hypertensive rat.' Biochemical Journal, 186,
       483-490.

1408. RAGOZIN, A.S., LANDESMAN-DWYER, S., and STREISSGUTH, A.P. (1978)
       'The relationship between mother's drinking habits and chil-
       dren's home environment.' In: Currents in Alcoholism.
       Volume 4. Ed. F.A. Seixas. New York: Grune and Stratton,
       pp. 39-49.

1409. RÄIHÄ, N.C.R., KOSKINEN, M., and PIKKARAINEN, P. (1967) 'De-
       velopmental changes in alcohol-dehydrogenase activity in
       rat and guinea-pig liver.' Biochemical Journal (London),
       103, 623-626.

1410. RAIVIO, K. and MÄENPÄÄ, P. (1979) 'Alkoholi ja sikiövauriot.'
       ['Alcohol and damage to the fetus.'] Katiloehti: Tidskrift
       for Barnmorskor, 84, 308-315.

1411. RAIVIO, K., and MÄENPÄÄ, P. (1979) 'Fetal alcohol syndrome.'
       Duodecim, 95, 357-363.

1412. RAMAN, G., PURANDARE, T.V., and MUNSHI, S.R. (1976) 'Sterility
       induced in male rats by injection of chemical agents into
       the vas deferens.' Andrologia, 8, 321-325.

1413. RAMILO, J., and HARRIS, V.J. (1979) 'Neuroblastoma in a child
       with the hydantoin and fetal alcohol syndrome: The radio-
       graphic features.' British Journal of Radiology, 52, 993-
       995.

1414. RANDALL, C.L. (1977) 'Teratogenic effects on in utero ethanol
       exposure.' In: Alcohol and Opiates: Neurochemical and
       Behavioral Mechanisms. Ed. K. Blum, D.L. Bard, and M.G. Ham-
       ilton. New York: Academic Press, pp. 91-107.

1415. RANDALL, C.L. (1977) 'Teratogenic effects of in utero ethanol
       exposure.' Paper presented at the Fetal Alcohol Syndrome
       Workshop, San Diego, California.

1416. RANDALL, C.L. (1979) 'Introduction to fetal alcohol syndrome.'
       Currents in Alcoholism. Volume 5. Ed. M. Galanter.
       New York: Grune and Stratton, pp. 119-121.

1417. RANDALL, C.L. (1981) 'Alcohol as a teratogen in animals.'
       In: Biomedical Processes and Consequences of Alcohol Use.
       Alcohol and Health Monograph No. 2. Rockville, Maryland:
       National Institute on Alcohol Abuse and Alcoholism (in
       press).

1418. RANDALL, C.L. (1981) 'Summary and recommendations: Animal re-
       search on alcohol and pregnancy.' Neurobehavioral Toxi-
       cology and Teratology, 3, 237-238.

1419. RANDALL, C.L., and BOGGAN, W.O. (1977) 'Neurochemical manifes-
       tations of prenatal ethanol exposure in rats.' Alcoholism:
       Clinical and Experimental Research, 1, 156 (abstract).

1420. RANDALL, C.L., and BOGGAN, W.O. (1978) 'Dysmorphy in DBA/2J
       mice prenatally exposed to ethanol.' Alcoholism: Clinical
       and Experimental Research, 2, 215 (abstract).

1421. RANDALL, C.L., and BOGGAN, W.O. (1979) 'Comparisons of alcohol
       preference between male, pregnant and non-pregnant female
       $C_{57}BL$ mice.' Alcoholism: Clinical and Experimental Re-
       search, 3, 191 (abstract).

1422. RANDALL, C.L., BOGGAN, W.O., and MOLONY-SINNOTT, V. (1980) 'Ef-
       fect of low-dose prenatal alcohol exposure on behavior and
       the response to alcohol.' Alcoholism: Clinical and Exper-
       imental Research, 4, 226 (abstract).

1423. RANDALL, C.L., BOGGAN, W.O., and SUTKER, P.B. (1980) 'Voluntary
       consumption of ethanol during pregnancy lactation and post-
       lactation in mice.' Drug and Alcohol Dependence, 6, 48.

1424. RANDALL, C.L., LOCHRY, E.A., HUGHES, S.S., and BOGGAN, W.O.
       (1980) 'Decreased ethanol consumption as a function of
       pregnancy and lactation in $C_{57}BL$ mice.' Pharmacology, Bio-
       chemistry, and Behavior, 13, Supplement 1, 149-153.

1425. RANDALL, C.L., LOCHRY, E.A., HUGHES, S.S., and SUTKER, P.B.
       (1981) 'The effect of ovariectomy and estrus cycle on sensi-
       tivity to acute alcohol challenge in C3H mice.' Alcoholism:
       Clinical and Experimental Research, 5, 164 (abstract).

1426. RANDALL, C.L., LOCHRY, E.A., MOSELEY, J.W., and SUTKER, P.B.
       (1981) 'Alcohol sensitivity in female mice: Effect of
       ovariectomy.' Pharmacology, Biochemistry, and Behavior, 15,
       191-195.

1427.   RANDALL, C.L., LOCHRY, E.A., and SUTKER, P.B.   (1981)   'Effects
        of acute alcohol exposure during selected days of gestation
        in C$_3$H mice.'   Teratology, 23, 57A (abstract).

1428.   RANDALL, C.L., and NOBLE, E.P.   (1980)   'Alcohol abuse and fetal
        growth and development.'   In: Advances in Substance Abuse,
        Behavioral and Biological Research: A Research Annual.
        Ed. N.K. Mello.   Greenwich, Connecticut: JAI Press,
        pp. 327-367.

1429.   RANDALL, C.L., and RILEY, E.P.   (1981)   'Prenatal alcohol ex-
        posure: Current issues and the status of animal research.'
        Neurobehavioral Toxicology and Teratology, 3, 111-115.

1430.   RANDALL, C.L., and TAYLOR, W.J.   (1979)   'Prenatal ethanol ex-
        posure in mice: Teratogenic effects.'   Teratology, 19,
        305-312.

1431.   RANDALL, C., TAYLOR, W.J., and TABAKOFF, B.   (1976)   'Ethanol as
        a teratogen.'   Paper presented at the Second International
        Symposium on Alcohol and Aldehyde Metabolizing Systems,
        Philadelphia.

1432.   RANDALL, C.L., TAYLOR, W.J., TABAKOFF, B., and WALKER, D.W.
        (1977)   'Ethanol as a teratogen.'   In: Alcohol and Aldehyde
        Metabolizing Systems.   Ed. R.G. Thurman, J.R. Williamson,
        H.R. Drott, and B. Chance.   New York: Academic Press,
        pp. 659-670.

1433.   RANDALL, C.L., TAYLOR, W.J., and WALKER, D.W.   (1977)   'Ethanol-
        induced malformations in mice.'   Alcoholism: Clinical and
        Experimental Research, 1, 219-223.

1434.   RASMUSSEN, B.B., and CHRISTENSEN, N.   (1978)   'Alkohol og foster-
        skader.'   ['Alcohol and fetal damage.']   Ugeskrift for
        Laeger (Copenhagen), 140, 282-284.

1435.   RASMUSSEN, B.B., and CHRISTENSEN, N.   (1980)   'Teratogenic effect
        of maternal alcohol consumption on the mouse fetus: A histo-
        pathological study.'   Acta Pathologica Microbiologica Scand-
        inavica, Section A, Pathology, 88, 285-289.

1436.   RATHOD, N.H., and THOMSON, I.G.   (1971)   'Women alcoholics; a
        clinical study.'   Quarterly Journal of Studies on Alcohol,
        32, 45-52.

1437.   RAWAT, A.K.   (1975)   'Effects of maternal ethanol consumption
        on the fetal and neonatal cerebral neurotransmitters.'
        In: The Role of Acetaldehyde in the Actions of Ethanol.
        Volume 23.   Ed. K.O. Lindros and C.J.P. Eriksson.   Helsinki:
        The Finnish Foundation for Alcohol Studies, pp. 159-176.

1438.   RAWAT, A.K.   (1975)   'Ribosomal protein synthesis in the fetal
        and neonatal rat brain as influenced by maternal ethanol
        consumption.'   Research Communications in Chemical Pathology
        and Pharmacology, 12, 723-732.

1439. RAWAT, A.K.   (1975)   'Ribosomal protein synthesis in the fetal
       brain as influenced by maternal ethanol consumption.'
       Federation Proceedings; Federation of American Societies for
       Experimental Biology, 34, 224.

1440. RAWAT, A.K.   (1976)   'Effect of maternal ethanol consumption
       on fetal hepatic metabolism in the rat.'   Annals of the
       New York Academy of Sciences, 273, 175-187.

1441. RAWAT, A.K.   (1976)   'Effect of maternal ethanol consumption on
       foetal and neonatal rat hepatic protein synthesis.'   Bio-
       chemical Journal (London), 160, 653-661.

1442. RAWAT, A.K.   (1976)   'Protein metabolism in fetal rat liver from
       chronic alcoholic mothers.'   In: Proteolysis and Physio-
       logical Regulation.   Ed. D.W. Ribbons and K. Brew.
       New York: Academic Press, p. 403.

1443. RAWAT, A.K.   (1977)   'Developmental changes in the brain levels
       of neurotransmitters as influenced by maternal ethanol con-
       sumption in the rat.'   Journal of Neurochemistry (London),
       28, 1175-1182.

1444. RAWAT, A.K.   (1978)   'Biochemical bases of cardiac anomalies in
       fetal alcohol syndrome.'   Federation Proceedings; Federation
       of American Societies for Experimental Biology, 37, 1351
       (abstract).

1445. RAWAT, A.K.   (1978)   'Effects of maternal ethanol consumption on
       hepatic lipid biosynthesis in foetal and neonatal rats.'
       Biochemical Journal, 174, 213-219.

1446. RAWAT, A.K.   (1978)   'Fetal alcohol syndrome; metabolic abnor-
       malities.'   Ohio State Medical Journal, 74, 109-111.

1447. RAWAT, A.K.   (1979)   'Derangement in cardiac protein metabolism
       in fetal alcohol syndrome.'   Research Communications in
       Chemical Pathology and Pharmacology, 25, 365-375.

1448. RAWAT, A.K.   (1979)   'Psychotropic drug metabolism in fetal alco-
       hol syndrome.'   Alcoholism: Clinical and Experimental Re-
       search, 3, 272 (abstract).

1449. RAWAT, A.K.   (1979)   'Psychotropic drug metabolism in fetal alco-
       hol syndrome.'   Third International Symposium on Alcohol and
       Aldehyde Metabolizing Systems, p. 20 (abstract).

1450. RAWAT, A.K.   (1980)   'Biochemical aspects of neuroteratogenic
       effects of ethanol.'   Neurobehavioral Toxicology, 2, 259-265.

1451. RAWAT, A.K.   (1980)   'Biochemical basis of neuroteratological
       effects of ethanol.'   Teratology, 21, 64A (abstract).

1452. RAWAT, A.K.   (1980)   'Development of histaminergic pathways in
       brain as influenced by maternal alcoholism.'   Research Com-
       munications in Chemical Pathology and Pharmacology, 27, 91-103.

1453. RAWAT, A.K. (1980) 'Neurotoxic effects of maternal alcoholism
       on the developing fetus and newborn.' Advances in Neuro-
       toxicology, Proceedings of the International Congress,
       pp. 155-163.

1454. RAWAT, A.K. (1980) 'Pharmacological and toxicological con-
       siderations in fetal alcohol syndrome.' In: Alcoholism:
       A Perspective. Ed. F.S. Messiha and G.S. Tyner. Westbury,
       New York: PJD Publications, pp. 149-176.

1455. RAWAT, A.K. (1980) 'Psychotropic drug metabolism in fetal alco-
       hol syndrome.' Advances in Experimental Medicine and Bio-
       logy, 132, 561-568.

1456. RAWAT, A.K. (1981) 'Ethanol and psychotropic drug interaction
       during pregnancy and lactation.' Biochemical Pharmacology,
       30, 2457-2460.

1457. RAWAT, A.K., and KUMAR, S. (1977) 'Effects of maternal ethanol
       consumption on the metabolism of dopamine in rat fetus and
       neonate.' Research Communications in Psychology, Psychiatry,
       and Behavior, 2, 117-129.

1458. REDMOND, G.P. (1979) 'Effect of drugs on intrauterine growth.'
       Clinical Perinatology, 6, 5-19.

1459. REDMOND, G.P. (1980) 'Effect of ethanol on pulsatile gonado-
       tropin secretion in the male rat.' Alcoholism: Clinical
       and Experimental Research, 4, 226 (abstract).

1460. REID, G.A. (1903) 'Human evolution; with especial reference to
       alcohol.' British Medical Journal (London), 2, 818-820.

1461. REIFF, J.S. (1980) 'Fetal alcohol syndrome.' Maryland State
       Medical Journal, 29, 20-21.

1462. REINHOLD, L., HÜTTEROTH, H., and SCHULTE-WISSERMANN, H. (1975)
       'Das fetale Alkohol-Syndrom: Fallbericht über 2 Geschwis-
       ter.' ['The fetal alcohol syndrome: Case report of two
       siblings.'] Münchener Medizinische Wochenschrift (Munich),
       117, 1731-1734.

1463. REISNER, S., and DAVIDOWITZ, M. (1979) 'Fetal alcohol syndrome.'
       [Editorial.] Harefuah, 97, 138-139.

1464. RENAUT, P. (1901) Contribution à l'étude de l'alcoolisme con-
       genital au point de vue experimental et clinique. [Contri-
       bution to the study of alcoholism from the experimental and
       clinical point of view.] Paris: Rousset.

1465. RIBAKOFF, F.Y. (1910) 'Heredity and alcoholism, statistical in-
       vestigations based on 2,000 cases.' Zhurnal Nevropatologii
       i Psikhiatrii imeni s s Korsakova (Moscow), 10, 338-348.

1466. RICE, C. (1979) 'Epidemiological analyses of FAS--nature, ex-
       tent, significance.' Paper presented at the Conference on
       Women and Alcohol, New York (February 14).

1467. RICHARDS, T.M. (1979) 'Working with disturbed children of an
       alcoholic mother.' Alcoholism: Clinical and Experimental
       Research, 3, 192 (abstract).

1468. RIDER, A.A. (1979) 'Adaptation to moderate ethanol intake as
       reflected in reproductive performance in the rat.' Nutri-
       tion Reports International, 19, 765-772.

1469. RIDGE, J.J. (1893) Alcohol and Public Health. London.

1470. RIDGE, J.J. (1898) 'The action of alcohol on frog's spawn.'
       Medical Temperance Review, 1, 14, 86.

1471. RILEY, E.P. (1978) 'Lack of response inhibition in rats pre-
       natally exposed to alcohol.' Paper presented at the Psycho-
       nomic Society Meeting, San Antonio, Texas.

1472. RILEY, E.P. (1980) 'Behavioral effects of exposure at different
       stages of gestation.' Paper presented at the Fetal Alcohol
       Syndrome Workshop, Seattle, Washington (May 2-4).

1473. RILEY, E.P. (1980) 'Fetal alcohol syndrome and fetal alcohol
       effects: An animal model.' Fifth Food and Drug Administra-
       tion Science Symposium on the Effects of Foods and Drugs on
       the Development and Function of the Nervous System.
       Ed. R.M. Gryder and V.H. Frankos. HHH Publication No. (FDA)
       80-1076.

1474. RILEY, E.P. (1980) 'Review of ethanol as a behavioral terato-
       gen.' Paper presented at the International Society for
       Developmental Psychobiology, Cincinnati, Ohio (November 8).

1475. RILEY, E.P. (1981) 'Differential tissue sensitivity to ethanol:
       A possible role in the etiology of fetal alcohol syndrome.'
       [Letter.] Substance and Alcohol Actions/Misuse, 2, 203-204.

1476. RILEY, E.P. (1981) 'Animal models of alcohol-induced behavioral
       teratology.' Teratology, 23, 57A (abstract).

1477. RILEY, E.P. (1981) 'Ethanol as a behavioral teratogen.' Alco-
       hol and Health Monograph, No. 2 (in press).

1478. RILEY, E.P. (1981) 'Ethanol as a behavioral teratogen: Animal
       studies.' Teratology, 23, 57A (abstract).

1479. RILEY, E.P., DRISCOLL, C., and CHEN, J.S. (1980) 'Instrumental
       runway and operant-DRL performance in rat offspring following
       prenatal alcohol-exposure.' Teratology, 21, 64A (abstract).

1480. RILEY, E.P., DRISCOLL, C.D., and CHEN, J.S. (1980) 'Passive
        avoidance performance in rats prenatally exposed to alcohol
        during different periods of gestation.' Paper presented
        at the Fetal Alcohol Syndrome Workshop, Seattle, Washington.

1481. RILEY, E.P., and LOCHRY, E.A. (1981) 'Genetic influences in
        the etiology of fetal alcohol syndrome.' In: Fetal Alco-
        hol Syndrome. Volume 3: Animal Studies. Ed. E.L. Abel.
        Boca Raton, Florida: CRC Press (in press).

1482. RILEY, E.P., LOCHRY, E.A., and SHAPIRO, N.R. (1979) 'Alcohol-
        induced behavioral teratogenesis: An animal model.' Paper
        presented at the American Psychological Convention, New York.

1483. RILEY, E.P., LOCHRY, E.A., and SHAPIRO, N.R. (1979) 'Growth
        deficits in rats after prenatal alcohol exposure.' Paper
        presented at the 87th Annual Convention of the American
        Psychological Association, New York.

1484. RILEY, E.P., LOCHRY, E.A., and SHAPIRO, N.R. (1979) 'Lack of
        response inhibition in rats prenatally exposed to alcohol.'
        Psychopharmacology (Berlin), 62, 47-52.

1485. RILEY, E.P., LOCHRY, E.A., and SHAPIRO, N.R. (1980) 'Alcohol-
        induced behavioral teratogenesis: An animal model.' In:
        Animal Models in Alcohol Research: Papers Presented at the
        International Conference on Animal Models in Alcohol Re-
        search, Helsinki, Finland (4-8 June, 1979). Ed. K. Eriks-
        son, J.D. Sinclair, and K. Kiianmaa. London and New York:
        Academic Press, pp. 393-399.

1486. RILEY, E.P., LOCHRY, E.A., SHAPIRO, N.R., and BALDWIN, J. (1979)
        'Response perseveration in rats exposed to alcohol pre-
        natally.' Pharmacology, Biochemistry, and Behavior, 10,
        255-259.

1487. RILEY, E.P., SHAPIRO, N.R., and LOCHRY, E.A. (1979) 'Nose-
        poking and head-dipping behaviors in rats prenatally ex-
        posed to ethanol.' Pharmacology, Biochemistry, and Behav-
        ior, 11, 513-519.

1488. RILEY, E.P., SHAPIRO, N.R., LOCHRY, E.A., and BROIDA, J.P. (1980)
        'Fixed-ratio performance and subsequent extinction in rats
        prenatally exposed to ethanol.' Physiological Psychology, 8,
        47-50.

1489. RIVARD, C. (1979) 'The fetal alcohol syndrome.' Journal of
        School Health, 49, 96-98.

1490. ROBE, L.B. (1977) Just So It's Healthy. Minneapolis, Minnesota:
        Comp Care Publications

1491. ROBE, L.B. (1981) 'If mama boozes, baby loses.' U.S. Journal of
        Drug and Alcohol Dependence, 4, 9.

1492.   ROBE, L.B., GROMISCH, D.S., and IOSUB, S.   (1980)   'Symptoms of
        neonatal ethanol withdrawal.'   Alcoholism: Clinical and
        Experimental Research, 4, 227 (abstract).

1493.   ROBE, L.B., ROBE, R.S., and WILSON, P.A.   (1979)   'Maternal heavy
        drinking related to delayed onset of daughters' menstru-
        ation.'   Alcoholism: Clinical and Experimental Research, 3,
        192 (abstract).

1494.   ROBE, L.B., ROBE, R.S., and WILSON, P.A.   (1980)   'Maternal heavy
        drinking related to delayed onset of daughters' menstru-
        ation.'   In: Currents in Alcoholism. Volume 7: Recent
        Advances in Research and Treatment. Ed. M. Galanter.
        New York: Grune and Stratton, pp. 515-520.

1495.   ROBINOVITCH, L.G.   (1901)   'Idiot and imbecile children; various
        causes of idiocy and imbecility; the relation of alcoholism
        in the parent to idiocy and imbecility of the offspring;
        a clinical study.'   Journal of Mental Pathology, 1, 14, 86-
        95.

1496.   ROBINOVITCH, L.G.   (1903)   'Infantile alcoholism.'   Quarterly
        Journal of Inebriety, 25, 231-236.

1497.   ROBINSON, R.O.   (1977)   'Fetal alcohol syndrome.'   Developmental
        Medicine and Child Neurobiology (London), 19, 538-540.

1498.   RODIN, A.E.   (1981)   'Infants and gin mania in 18th-century Lon-
        don.'   Journal of the American Medical Association, 245,
        1237-1239.

1499.   ROE, D.A.   (1976)   'Fetal malnutrition, abnormal development,
        and growth retardation.'   In: Drug Induced Nutritional
        Deficiencies. Westport, Connecticut: Avi Publishing Com-
        pany, pp. 187-201.

1500.   ROELS, H., HUBERMONT, G., BUCHET, J.P., and LAUWERYS, R.   (1978)
        'Placental transfer of lead, mercury, cadmium, and carbon
        monoxide in women. III. Factors influencing the accumula-
        tion of heavy metals in the placenta and the relationship
        between metal concentration in the placenta and in maternal
        and cord blood.'   Environmental Research, 16, 236-247.

1501.   ROHNER, S.W.   (1980)   'Fetal alcohol effects linked to moderate
        drinking levels.'   Maryland State Medical Journal, 29, 26-
        27.

1502.   RONNING, G.   (1981)   'Fetal alcohol syndrome cause for alarm.'
        Alberta Alcoholism and Drug Abuse Commission, 1, n. pag.

1503.   ROOT, A.W., REITER, E.O., ANDRIOLA, M., and DUCKETT, G.   (1975)
        'Hypothalamic-pituitary function in the fetal alcohol syn-
        drome.'   Journal of Pediatrics, 87, 585-588.

1504.   ROSANELLI, K.   (1977)   'Schäden bei Kindern von Müttern mit
        chronischem Alkoholismus (Alkoholembryopathie).'   ['Damage
        to children of chronically alcoholic mothers (alcohol embryo-
        pathy).']   Wiener Medizinische Wochenschrift (Vienna), 127,
        544-546.

1505.   ROSE, J.C.   (1980)   'Alcohol and fetal endocrine function.'
        Paper presented at the Fetal Alcohol Syndrome Workshop,
        Seattle, Washington (May 2-4).

1506.   ROSE, J.C., MEIS, P.J., and CASTRO, M.I.   (1981)   'Alcohol and
        fetal endocrine function.'   Neurobehavioral Toxicology and
        Teratology, 3, 105-110.

1507.   ROSE, J.C., STRANDHOY, J.W., and MEIS, P.J.   (1980)   'Acute and
        chronic effects of maternal ethanol administration in the
        ovine maternal-fetal unit.'   Pharmacology, Biochemistry, and
        Behavior, 12, 329 (abstract).

1508.   ROSELLINI, R.A., RILEY, E.P., and HUBNER, C.B.   (1981)   'Pav-
        lovian fear conditioning in rats prenatally exposed to
        alcohol.'   Alcoholism: Clinical and Experimental Research,
        5, 165 (abstract).

1509.   ROSENAU, M.J.   (1916)   Preventive Medicine and Hygiene.
        New York: Appleton.

1510.   ROSENBAUM, B.   (1958)   'Married women alcoholics at the Washing-
        tonian Hospital.'   Quarterly Journal of Studies on Alcohol,
        19, 79-89.

1511.   ROSENLICHT, J. MURPHY, J.B., and MALONEY, P.L.   (1979)   'Fetal
        alcohol syndrome.'   Oral Surgery, Oral Medicine, Oral Path-
        ology, 47, 8-10.

1512.   ROSETT, H.L.   (1974)   'Maternal alcoholism and intellectual de-
        velopment of offspring.'   Lancet (London), 2, 218.

1513.   ROSETT, H.L.   (1976)   'Effects of alcohol on offspring, including
        the fetal alcohol syndrome.'   Contract NIA 76-25 (P).

1514.   ROSETT, H.L.   (1976)   'The effects of maternal drinking on child
        development: An introductory review.'   Annals of the
        New York Academy of Sciences, 273, 115-117.

1515.   ROSETT, H.L.   (1976)   'The prenatal clinic: A site for alco-
        holism prevention and treatment.'   Paper presented at the
        7th Annual Medical-Scientific Session of the National Alco-
        holism Forum, Washington, D.C.

1516.   ROSETT, H.L.   (1978)   'Effects of ethanol on offspring: Including
        the fetal alcohol syndrome.'   Third Special Report to the
        U.S. Congress on "Alcohol and Health."   Department of Health,
        Education, and Welfare, pp. 171-193.

1517. ROSETT, H.L.   (1978)   'Therapy of heavy drinking pregnancy.'
       Paper presented at Fetal Alcohol Syndrome Symposium, Ann Ar-
       bor, Michigan.

1518. ROSETT, H.L.   (1979)   'Clinical pharmacology of the fetal alcohol
       syndrome.' In: Biochemistry and Pharmacology of Ethanol.
       Volume 2. Ed. E. Majchrowicz and E.P. Noble. New York and
       London: Plenum Press, pp. 485-509.

1519. ROSETT, H.L.   (1979)   'Effects of alcohol on fetus and off-
       spring.' In: Research Advances in Alcohol and Drug Prob-
       lems. Volume 5. Ed. P.J. Kalande. New York: Plenum
       Press (in press).

1520. ROSETT, H.L.   (1980)   'Biochemical pharmacology of the fetal
       alcohol syndrome.' In: Biochemical Pharmacology of Ethanol.
       Ed. E. Majchrowicz and E.P. Noble. New York: Plenum Press.

1521. ROSETT, H.L.   (1980)   'A clinical perspective of the fetal alco-
       hol syndrome.' [Editorial.] Alcoholism: Clinical and Ex-
       perimental Research, 4, 119-122.

1522. ROSETT, H.L.   (1980)   'Needed: Experimental research to answer
       clinical questions.' Teratology, 21, 65A (abstract).

1523. ROSETT, H.L.   (1980)   'Remarks on methodology: NIAAA prospective
       studies.' Paper presented at the Fetal Alcohol Syndrome
       Workshop, Seattle, Washington (May 2-4).

1524. ROSETT, H.L.   (1980)   'The effects of alcohol on the fetus and
       offspring.' In: Alcohol and Drug Problems in Women.
       Ed. O.J. Kalant. New York: Plenum Publishing Company,
       pp. 595-652.

1525. ROSETT, H.L.   (1981)   'Psychiatric aspects of the fetal alcohol
       syndrome.' Paper presented at the World Psychiatric Meeting,
       New York (October 31-November 1).

1526. ROSETT, H.L.   (1981)   'Summary and recommendations: NIAAA pro-
       spective fetal alcohol studies.' Neurobehavioral Toxicology
       and Teratology, 3, 243-245.

1527. ROSETT, H.L., and OUELLETTE, E.M.   (1976)   'Effects of maternal
       drinking on offspring.' In: The Patient with Alcoholism and
       Other Drug Dependencies. Ed. C. Whitfield and K. Williams.
       Springfield, Illinois: Southern Illinois University Press.

1528. ROSETT, H.L., OUELLETTE, E.M., and WEINER, L.   (1976)   'A pilot
       prospective study of the fetal alcohol syndrome at the Bos-
       ton City Hospital. Part I: Maternal drinking.' Annals of
       the New York Academy of Sciences, 273, 118-122.

1529. ROSETT, H.L., OUELLETTE, E.M., WEINER, L., and OWENS, E.   (1977)
       'The prenatal clinic: A site for alcoholism prevention
       and treatment.' In: Currents in Alcoholism. Volume 1.
       Ed. F.A. Seixas. New York: Grune and Stratton, pp. 419-430.

1530.   ROSETT, H.L., OUELLETTE, E.M., WEINER, L., and OWENS, E.   (1978)
        'Therapy of heavy drinking during pregnancy.' American
        Journal of Obstetrics and Gynecology, 51, 41-46.

1531.   ROSETT, H.L., and SANDER, L.W.   (1979) 'Effects of maternal
        drinking on neonatal morphology and state regulation.'
        In: Handbook of Infant Development. Ed. J.D. Osofsky.
        New York: John Wiley and Sons, pp. 809-836.

1532.   ROSETT, H.L., SNYDER, P., SANDER, L.W., LEE, A., COOK, P.,
        WEINER, L., and GOULD, J.   (1979) 'Effects of maternal
        drinking on neonate state regulation.' Developmental
        Medicine and Child Neurology (London), 21, 464-473.

1533.   ROSETT, H.L., and WEINER, L.   (1975) 'Pregnancy and alcohol
        use: A Boston City Hospital survey.' Paper presented at
        the Symposium on the Consequences of Alcohol and Drug Abuse
        during Pregnancy on the Mother and her Offspring, New York.

1534.   ROSETT, H.L. and WEINER, L.   (1978) 'Reduction of alcohol con-
        sumption during pregnancy with benefits to the newborn.'
        Alcoholism: Clinical and Experimental Research, 2, 202
        (abstract).

1535.   ROSETT, H.L., and WEINER, L.   (1980) 'Adverse effects of heavy
        drinking during pregnancy: Including the fetal alcohol
        syndrome.' In: Phenomenology and Treatment of Alcoholism.
        Ed. W.E. Fann, I. Karacan, A.D. Pokorny, and R.L. Williams.
        New York: SP Medical and Scientific Books, pp. 139-149.

1536.   ROSETT, H.L., and WEINER, L.   (1980) 'Clinical and experimental
        perspectives on prevention of the fetal alcohol syndrome.'
        Neurobehavioral Toxicology, 2, 267-270.

1537.   ROSETT, H.L., and WEINER, L.   (1980) 'Prevention of the fetal
        alcohol syndrome.' Teratology, 21, 65a (abstract).

1538.   ROSETT, H.L., and WEINER, L.   (1981) 'Identifying and treating
        pregnant patients at risk from alcohol.' Canadian Medical
        Association Journal, 125, 149-158.

1539.   ROSETT, H.L., WEINER, L., and EDELIN, K.C.   (1981) 'Behavioral
        measurement in evaluation of fetal alcohol education for
        physicians.' Alcoholism: Clinical and Experimental Re-
        search, 5, 165 (abstract).

1540.   ROSETT, H.L., WEINER, L., and EDELIN, K.C.   (1981) 'Strategies
        for prevention of fetal alcohol effects.' Obstetrics and
        Gynecology, 57, 1-7.

1541.   ROSETT, H.L., WEINER, L., ZUCKERMAN, B., MC KINLAY, S., and
        EDELIN, K.C.   (1980) 'Reduction of alcohol consumption
        during pregnancy with benefits to the newborn.' Alcoholism:
        Clinical and Experimental Research, 4, 178-184.

1542.   ROSMAN, N.P., and MALONE, M.J.   (1976)   'An experimental study
        of the fetal alcohol syndrome.'   Neurology, 26, 365.

1543.   ROSMAN, N.P., and MALONE, M.J.   (1977)   'Reversal of delayed
        myelinogenesis in the fetal alcohol syndrome.'   Neurology,
        27, 369.

1544.   ROSMAN, N.P., and MALONE, M.J.   (1979)   'Spontaneous reversal of
        delayed myelinogenesis in experimental fetal alcohol syn-
        drome.'   Neurology, 29, 543.

1545.   ROSS, D.   (1977)   'Studies on the fetal alcohol syndrome using
        the rabbit as a maternal fetal model.'   Paper presented at
        the Fetal Alcohol Syndrome Workshop, San Diego, California.

1546.   ROST, E., and WOLF, G.   (1925)   'Zur Frage des Beeinflussung den
        Nachkommenschaft durch Alkohol im Tiefversuch.'   ['The prob-
        lem of the influence of alcohol on the offspring in ani-
        mals.']   Archiv für Hygiene, 95, 140-153.

1547.   ROWAN, J.J.   (1976)   'Excretion of drugs in milk.'   [Letter.]
        Pharmaceutical Journal, 217, 184-186.

1548.   ROWE, P.H., RACEY, P.A., and SHENTON, J.C., ELLWOOD, M., and
        LEHANE, J.   (1974)   'Effects of acute administration of al-
        cohol and barbiturates on plasma luteinizing hormone and
        testosterone in man.'   Journal of Endocrinology (London),
        63, 50P.

1549.   RUBIN, E., LIEBER, C.S., ALTMAN, K., GORDON, G.G., and SOUTHERN,
        A.L.   (1976)   'Prolonged ethanol consumption increases tes-
        tosterone metabolism in the liver.'   Science, 191, 563-564.

1550.   RUBIN, H.B., and HENSON, D.E.   (1976)   'Effects of alcohol on
        male sexual responding.'   Psychopharmacology (Berlin), 47,
        123-134.

1551.   RUSH, B.   (1787)   An Enquiry into the Effects of Spirituous
        Liquors upon the Human Body and their Influence upon the
        Happiness of Society.   Philadelphia: Thomas Dobson.

1552.   RUSH, B.   (1812)   An Inquiry into the Effects of Ardent Spirits
        upon the Human Body and Mind; with an Account of the Means
        of Preventing, and of the Remedies for Curing Them.   Boston:
        Manning and Loring.

1553.   RUSSELL, M.   (1975)   'Incidence of conditions associated with the
        fetal alcohol syndrome in children born to women with a his-
        tory of alcohol abuse.'   American Journal of Epidemiology,
        102, 437.

1554.   RUSSELL, M.   (1977)   'Intrauterine growth in infants born to
        women with alcohol-related psychiatric diagnoses.'   Alco-
        holism: Clinical and Experimental Research, 1, 225-231.

1555. RUSSELL, M. (1980) 'Obstetric and gynecologic problems, depres-
            sion, and alcohol use.' Paper presented at the 11th Annual
            Forum, Seattle, Washington (May 2-4).

1556. RUSSELL, M. (1980) 'Obstetric and gynecologic (ob-gyn) prob-
            lems, depression, and alcohol use.' Alcoholism: Clinical
            and Experimental Research, 4, 227 (abstract).

1557. RUSSELL, M. (1980) 'The impact of alcohol-related birth de-
            fects (ARBD) on New York State.' Neurobehavioral Toxicology,
            2, 277-283.

1558. RUSSELL, M. (1981) 'Screening for alcohol-related problems in
            obstetric and gynecologic patients.' In: Fetal Alcohol
            Syndrome. Volume 2: Human Studies. Ed. E.L. Abel.
            Boca Raton, Florida: CRC Press (in press).

1159. RUSSELL, M. (1981) 'The epidemiology of alcohol-related birth
            defects.' In: Fetal Alcohol Syndrome. Volume 2: Human
            Studies. Ed. E.L. Abel. Boca Raton, Florida: CRC Press
            (in press).

1560. RUSSELL, M., and BIGLER, L. (1977) 'Screening for alcohol-
            related problems in an outpatient ob-gyn clinic.' Paper
            presented at the Annual Meeting of the Society for Epidemio-
            logic Research, Seattle, Washington.

1561. RUSSELL, M., and BIGLER, L. (1977) 'Validation of a procedure
            to screen for alcohol-related problems in an ob-gyn popu-
            lation.' Paper presented at the 105th Annual Meeting of the
            American Public Health Association, Washington, D.C. (Octo-
            ber 30-November 3).

1562. RUSSELL, M., and BIGLER, L.R. (1979) 'Alcohol and other psycho-
            active drug intake among obstetric and gynecology patients.'
            Paper presented at the National Alcoholism Forum of the
            National Council on Alcoholism, Washington, D.C. (April).

1563. RUSSELL, M., and BIGLER, L.R. (1979) 'Screening for alcohol-
            related problems in an outpatient obstetric-gynecologic
            clinic.' American Journal of Obstetrics and Gynecology,
            34, 4-12.

1564. RUSSELL, M., LYONS, J.P., and BROWN, J. (1981) 'Development of
            a self-administered questionnaire to screen for alcohol-
            related problems in women.' Paper presented at the 12th
            Annual Medical-Scientific Conference of the National Council
            on Alcoholism, New Orleans, Louisiana (April 12-15).

1565. RUSSELL, M., LYONS, J.P., and BROWN, J. (1981) 'Development of
            a self-administered questionnaire to screen for alcohol-
            related problems in women.' Alcoholism: Experimental and
            Clinical Research, 5, 166 (abstract).

1566.   RYBACK, R.S.   (1977)   'Chronic alcohol consumption and menstru-
        ation.'   [Letter.]   Journal of the American Medical Assoc-
        iation, 238, 2143.

S

1567. SAGHIR, M.T., ROBINS, E., WALBRAN, B., and GENTRY, K.A. (1970) 'Homosexuality. IV. Psychiatric disorders and disability in the female homosexual.' American Journal of Psychiatry, 127, 147-154.

1568. ST. ALBIN GREENE, D. (1976) 'Alcoholism: A threat to the unborn.' National Observer, June 12.

1569. SALEEBY, C.W. (1909) 'Alcoholism and eugenics.' British Journal of Inebriety, 7, 7-20.

1570. SAMAILLE-VILLETTE, C.H., and SAMAILLE, P.-P. (1976) 'Le syndrome d'alcoolisme foetal. À propos de 47 observations.' ['Fetal alcohol syndrome. Report of 47 cases.'] Thèse de médecine, Lille.

1571. SAMAILLE-VILLETTE, C.H., and SAMAILLE, P.-P. (1977) 'Le syndrome d'alcoolisme foetal.' ['The fetal alcohol syndrome.'] Journées Nationales de Neonatologie (Paris), 21, 37-43.

1572. SAMOSHKINA, N.A. (1964) 'Vulnerability of rat embryos to external agents in the preimplantation period of development.' [In Russian.] Doklady Akademii Nauk SSSR, 154, 484-487.

1573. SAMSON, H.H. (1979) 'Effect of chronic maternal ethanol consumption induced by psychogenic polydipsia upon fetal development.' Alcoholism: Clinical and Experimental Research, 3, 194 (abstract).

1574. SAMSON, H.H. (1981) 'Maternal ethanol consumption and fetal development in the rat: A comparison of ethanol exposure techniques.' Alcoholism: Clinical and Experimental Research, 5, 67-74.

1575. SAMSON, H.H., and DIAZ, J. (1980) 'Microencephaly resulting from maternal and neonatal ethanol exposure in the rat.' Alcoholism: Clinical and Experimental Research, 4, 228 (abstract).

1576. SAMSON, H.H., and DIAZ, J. (1981) 'Altered development of brain by neonatal ethanol exposure: Zinc levels during and after exposure.' Alcoholism: Clinical and Experimental Research, 5, 563-569.

1577. SAMSON, H.H., and DIAZ, J. (1981) 'Effects of neonatal ethanol exposure on brain development in rodents.' In: Fetal Alcohol Syndrome. Volume 3: Animal Studies. Ed. E.L. Abel. Boca Raton, Florida: CRC Press (in press).

1578. SAMSON, H.H., and DIAZ, J. (1981) 'Neonatal microcephaly induced by ethanol: Role of Zn.' Alcoholism: Clinical and Experimental Research, 5, 167 (abstract).

1579. SAMSON, H.H., WATERMAN, D.L. and WOODS, S.C. (1979) 'Effect of acute ethanol exposure upon fetal development in the rat.' Physiological Psychology, 7, 311-314.

1580. SANDBERG, D.H. (1961) 'Drugs in pregnancy: Their effects on the fetus and newborn.' California Medicine, 94, 287-291.

1581. SANDER, L.W., SNYDER, P.A., ROSETT, H.L., LEE, A., GOULD, J.B., and OUELLETTE, E.M. (1977) 'Effects of alcohol intake during pregnancy in newborn state regulation: A progress report.' Alcoholism: Clinical and Experimental Research, 1, 233-241.

1582. SANDMAIER, M. (1980) The Invisible Alcoholics: Women and Alcohol Abuse in America. New York: McGraw-Hill.

1583. SANDOR, G.G.S., SMITH, D.F., and MAC LEOD, P.M. (1980) 'Cardiac malformations in the foetal alcohol syndrome.' Clinical Research, 28, 118a (abstract).

1584. SANDOR, G.G.S., SMITH, D.F., and MAC LEOD, P.M. (1981) 'Cardiac malformations in the fetal alcohol syndrome.' Journal of Pediatrics, 98, 771-773.

1585. SANDOR, S. (1968) 'The influence of aethyl-alcohol on the developing chick embryo. II.' Revue Roumaine d'Embryologie et de Cytologie, Serie d'Embryologie (Bucharest), 5, 167-171.

1586. SANDOR, S. (1979) 'The prenatal noxious effect of ethanol.' Revue Roumaine de Morphologie, Embryologie et de Physiologie (Bucharest), 25, 211-223.

1587. SANDOR, S., and AMELS, D. (1968) 'The action of aethanol on the praenatal development of albino rats (an attempt of multiphasic screening).' Revue Roumaine d'Embryologie et de Cytologie, Serie d'Embryologie (Bucharest), 8, 105-118.

1588. SANDOR, S., CHECIU, M., FAZAKAS-TODEA, I., and G'ARBAN, Z. (1980) 'The effect of ethanol upon early development in mice and rats. I. In vivo effect upon preimplantation and early postimplantation stages.' Morphology and Embryology (Bucharest), 26, 265-274.

1589.   SANDOR, S., and ELIAS, S.   (1968)   'The influence of aethyl-
        alcohol on the development of the chick embryo.'   Revue
        Roumaine d'Embryologie et de Cytologie, Serie d'Embryologie
        (Bucharest), 5, 51-76.

1590.   SANDOR, S., and ELIAS, S.   (1968)   'The influence of aethyl-
        alcohol on the development of the chick embryo.   II.'   Revue
        Roumaine d'Embryologie et de Cytologie, Serie d'Embryologie
        (Bucharest), 5, 167-171.

1591.   SANDOR, S., FAZAKAS-TODEA, I., and CHECIU, M.   (1980)   'The ef-
        fect of ethanol upon early development in mice and rats.
        II. In vitro effect upon early postimplantation rat embryos.'
        Revue Roumaine de Morphologie, Embryologie et de Physiologie
        (Bucharest), 26, 315-320.

1592.   SANTOLAYA, J.M., MARTINEZ, G., GOROSTIZA, E., AIZPIRI, J., and
        HERNANDEZ, M.   (1978)   'Alcoholismo fetal.'   ['Fetal alcohol
        syndrome.']   Drogalcohol, 3, 183-192.

1593.   SAPEIKA, J.   (1947)   'The excretion of drugs in human milk: A
        review.'   Journal of Obstetrics and Gynecology of the British
        Empire, 54, 426-431.

1594.   SATKOVÁ, V., and BRÄUEROVÁ, E.   (1979)   'Děti s nočním pomočováním
        z rodin alkoholiků.'   ['Nocturnal enuresis in children from
        alcoholic families.]   Protialkoholiky Obzor (Bratislava),
        14, 123-128.

1595.   SAUL, G.   (1959)   'Blockade of ovulation in the rabbit by intox-
        icating doses of ethyl alcohol.'   Anatomical Record, 133,
        332 (abstract).

1596.   SAULE, H.   (1974)   'Fetales Alkohol-Syndrom: Ein Fallbericht.'
        ['Fetal alcohol syndrome: A case.']   Klinische Pädiatrie
        (Stuttgart), 186, 452-455.

1597.   SAXEN, I.   (1975)   'Epidemiology of cleft lip and palate: An at-
        tempt to rule out chance correlations.'   British Journal of
        Preventive Social Medicine, 29, 103-110.

1598.   SAXON, I.   (1975)   'Etiological variables in oral clefts.'   Pro-
        ceedings of the Finnish Dental Society, 71, Supplement,
        3-40.

1599.   SCHAEFER, O.   (1962)   'Alcoholic withdrawal syndrome in a newborn
        infant of a Yukon Indian mother.'   Canadian Medical Assoc-
        iation Journal (Toronto), 87, 1333-1334.

1600.   SCHANBERG, S.M.   (1979)   'Neurotropic drugs: Biogenic amines and
        brain function.'   Psychopharmacology Bulletin, NIMH, 15,
        56-57.

1601. SCHAPOSNIK, F., SALVIOLI, M.V., CAPUTO, C.H., and CASTELLETO, R.
        (1978) 'Alteraciones histopatológicas testiculares en el
        alcoholismo crónico.' ['Testicular histopathological
        changes in chronic alcoholism.'] Revista Clinica Espanola,
        150, 35-38.

1602. SCHARLIEB, M. (1913) 'Alcohol and the child-bearing woman.'
        British Journal of Inebriety, 11, 62-66.

1603. SCHEID, R. (1975) 'Changes in sexual performance due to liver
        disease.' Medical Aspects of Human Sexuality, 19, 67-79.

1604. SCHEINER, A.P., DONOVAN, C.M., and BARTOSHESKY, L.E. (1979)
        'Fetal alcohol syndrome in child whose parents had stopped
        drinking.' Lancet (London), 1, 1077-1078.

1605. SCHENKER, S. (1980) 'Pathogenic mechanisms of FAS.' Paper pre-
        sented at the Fetal Alcohol Syndrome Workshop, Seattle,
        Washington (May 2-4).

1606. SCHEPPE, K.J. (1977) 'Alkohol-Embryopathie. Zur verschiedenen
        Aldiagnoses pra- und postnatal Retardierter.' ['Alcohol
        embryopathy. Different pre- and postnatal retardation diag-
        noses.'] Pädiatrische Praxis, 18, 207-208.

1607. SCLARE, A.B. (1980) 'The foetal alcohol syndrome.' In: Camber-
        well Council on Alcoholism: Women and Alcohol. New York:
        Tavistock Publications, pp. 53-66.

1608. SCHMID, F. (1977) 'Alkohol-Embryo-Fetopathie.' ['Alcoholic
        embryofetal pathology.'] Fortschritte der Medizin (Munich),
        95, 2003-2005.

1609. SCHMIDT-MATTHIESEN, H. (1979) 'Medikamentöse Methoden.' ['Abor-
        tion by medication.'] Archives of Gynecology, 228, 365-378.

1610. SCHREIBER, R.A. (1979) 'Induction of susceptibility to audio-
        genic seizures by ethanol during a critical period of devel-
        opment.' Paper presented at the International Society for
        Developmental Psychobiology, Atlanta, Georgia (November).

1611. SCHREINER, W.E. (1977) 'The fetus at risk; fetal growth retard-
        ation.' Praxis (Bern), 66, 387-392.

1612. SCHUCKIT, M.A. (1972) 'Sexual disturbance in the woman alco-
        holic.' Medical Aspects of Human Sexuality, 6, 44-62.

1613. SCHULSINGER, F. (1980) 'Biological psychopathology.' Annual Re-
        view of Psychology, 31, 583-606.

1614. SCHWEIGHOFER, A. (1912) 'Alkohol und Nachkommenschaft.' ['Al-
        cohol and offspring.'] Österreichische Sanitätswesen
        (Vienna), 24, 517, 543, 567.

1615.   SCHWETZ, B.A., LEONG, B.K., and STAPLES, R.E. (1975) 'Tera-
        tology studies on inhaled carbon monoxide and imbibed
        ethanol in laboratory animals.' Teratology, 11, 33A (ab-
        stract).

1616.   SCHWETZ, B.A., SMITH, F.A., and STAPLES, R.E. (1978) 'Terato-
        genic potential of ethanol in mice, rats, and rabbits.'
        Teratology, 18, 385-392.

1617.   SCIANARO, L., PRUSEK, W., and LOIODICE, G. (1978) 'La sindrome
        del feto alcolizzato: Osservazioni cliniche.' ['The fetal
        alcohol syndrome: Clinical observations.'] Minerva
        Pediatrica (Torino), 30, 1585-1588.

1618.   SEDGEWICK, J. (1725) A New Treatise on Liquors, Wherein the Use
        and Abuse of Wine, Malt-Drinks, Water & C. are Particularly
        Considered in Many Diseases, Constitutions and Ages; with
        the Proper Manner of Using Them, Hot, or Cold, Either as
        Physick, Diet or Bath. . . . London: Charles Rivington.

1619.   SEELER, R.A., ISRAEL, J.N., ROYAL, J.E., KAYE, C.I., RAO, S., and
        ABULABAN, M. (1979) 'Ganglioneuroblastoma and fetal hydan-
        toin alcohol syndromes.' Pediatrics, 63, 524-527.

1620.   SEGAL, D.J. (1973-1974) 'Smoking, drinking, and your baby's
        mental health.' Mental Retardation Bulletin, 2, 64-67.

1621.   SEIDENBERG, J., and MAJEWSKI, F. (1978) 'Zur Häufigkeit der
        Alkoholembryopathie in den verschiedenen Phasen der mütter-
        lichen Alkoholkrankheit.' ['On the frequency of alcohol
        embryopathy in the different phases of maternal alcoholism.']
        Suchtgefahren (Hamburg), 24, 63-75.

1622.   SEIDLER, G. (1980) 'When considering pregnancy forget all about
        alcohol.' Focus on Alcohol and Drug Issues, 3, 20.

1623.   SEIXAS, F.A. (1977) 'The fetal alcohol syndrome.' [Editorial
        comment.] Alcoholism: Clinical and Experimental Research,
        1, 191-192.

1624.   SEIXAS, F.A. (1977) 'The fetal alcohol syndrome: A seminar.'
        [Editorial.] Alcoholism: Clinical and Experimental Re-
        search, 1, 217.

1625.   SEIXAS, F.A. (1979) 'Fetal alcohol syndrome and the year of the
        child.' Toxicomanies (Quebec), 12, 319-329.

1626.   SEMCZUK, M. (1978) 'Further investigations on the ultrastruc-
        ture of spermatozoa in chronic alcoholics.' Zeitschrift
        für Mikroskopisch-Anatomische Forschung, 92, 494-508.

1627.   SEMCZUK, M. (1978) 'Morphological research on the male gonad
        in long-lasting alcoholization of rats.' Gegenbaurs Mor-
        phologisches Jahrbuch, 124, 546-558.

1628. SEMCZUK, M. (1978) 'Ocena plemników szczurów poddanych przew-
       lekłej intoksykacji alkoholem etylowym.' ['Evaluation of
       rat sperm following chronic alcohol intoxication.'] Ginekologia
       Polska, 49, 955-961.

1629. SEMCZUK, M. (1979) '3-beta-hydroxysteroid dehydrogenase activ-
       ity and the morphological structure of Leydig's cells in
       white rat testicles under conditions of longlasting
       alcohol intoxication.' Materia Medica Polona, 11, 132-138.

1630. SEMCZUK, M., ŻRUBEK, H., and CZAJKA, R. (1978) 'Dalsze badania
       nad morfologią nasienia meżczyzn dotknietych przewlekłym
       alkoholizmem.' ['Morphology of sperm in chronic alco-
       holics.'] Polski Tygodnik Lekarski (Warsaw), 33, 961-964.

1631. SENSEMANN, L.A. (1976) 'The fetal alcohol syndrome.' Report of
       the Second World Congress for the Prevention of Alcoholism
       and Drug Dependency, Acapulco, Mexico (August 22-27).

1632. SEPPÄLÄ, M., RÄIHÄ, N.C., and TAMMINEN, V. (1971) 'Ethanol
       elimination in a mother and her premature twins.' Lancet
       (London), 1, 1188-1189.

1633. SEWARD, B. (1980) 'Education on the fetal alcoholism syndrome.'
       Seminar moderated at the National Council on Alcohol Con-
       ference, Seattle, Washington.

1634. SHANSKE, A.L., and KAZI, R. (1980) 'Prevalence of the fetal
       alcohol syndrome in a developmental clinic population.'
       American Journal of Human Genetics, 32, 128A (abstract).

1635. SHAPIRO, N.R., LOCHRY, E.A., and RILEY, E.P. (1979) 'Nose-
       poking behavior in rats prenatally exposed to alcohol.'
       Paper presented at the Eastern Psychological Association,
       50th Annual Meeting, Philadelphia, Pennsylvania.

1636. SHARMA, S.C., and CHAUDHURY, R.R. (1970) 'Studies on mating.
       Part II: The effect of ethanol on sperm transport and
       ovulation in successfully mated rabbits.' Indian Journal of
       Medical Research (New Delhi), 58, 501-504.

1637. SHAYWITZ, B.A. (1976) 'A syndrome resembling minimal brain
       dysfunction in rat pups born to alcoholic mothers.' Paper
       presented at the Fetal Alcohol Syndrome Workshop, San Diego,
       California.

1638. SHAYWITZ, B.A. (1977) 'A syndrome resembling minimum brain dys-
       function in rat pups born to alcoholic mothers.' NIAAA-
       sponsored Fetal Alcohol Syndrome Workshop, San Diego, Cal-
       ifornia.

1639. SHAYWITZ, B.A. (1978) 'Fetal alcohol syndrome: An ancient
       problem rediscovered.' Drug Therapy (Hospital), Vol. ?
       53-60.

1640.   SHAYWITZ, B.A., and GRIFFIETH, A.B.   (1977)   'Hyperactivity and cognitive deficits in developing rat pups born to alcoholic mothers: An experimental model of the fetal alcohol syndrome.'   Paper presented at the NIAAA Fetal Alcohol Syndrome Workshop, San Diego, California.

1641.   SHAYWITZ, B.A., GRIFFIETH, G.G., and WARSHAW, J.B.   (1979) 'Hyperactivity and cognitive deficits in developing rat pups born to alcoholic mothers: An experimental model of the expanded fetal alcohol syndrome (EFAS).'   Neurobehavioral Toxicology, 1, 113-122.

1642.   SHAYWITZ, B.A., KLOPPER, J.H., and GORDON, J.W.   (1976)   'A syndrome resembling minimal brain dysfunction (MBD) in rat pups born to alcoholic mothers.'   Pediatric Research, 10, 451 (abstract).

1643.   SHAYWITZ, S.E.   (1981)   'Attention deficit syndrome in children born to alcoholic mothers.'   [Letter.]   Journal of Pediatrics, 98, 671.

1644.   SHAYWITZ, S.E., COHEN, D.J., and SHAYWITZ, B.A.   (1978)   'The expanded fetal alcohol syndrome (EFAS)--Behavioral and learning deficits in children with normal intelligence.' Pediatric Research, 12, 375.

1645.   SHAYWITZ, S.E., COHEN, D.J., and SHAYWITZ, B.A.   (1980)   'Behavior and learning deficits in children of normal intelligence born to alcoholic mothers.'   Journal of Pediatrics, 96, 978-982.

1646.   SHELDON, C.H., and BORS, E.   (1948)   'Subarachnoid alcohol block in paraplegia: Its beneficial effect on mass reflexes and bladder dysfunction.'   Journal of Neurosurgery, 5, 385-391.

1647.   SHERFEY, M.J.   (1955)   'Psychopathology and character structure in chronic alcoholism.'   In: Etiology of Chronic Alcoholism.   Ed. O. Diethelm.   Springfield, Illinois: Thomas Publishing Company, pp. 16-42.

1648.   SHERWIN, B.T., and JACOBSON, S.   (1979)   'A rat model for the fetal alcohol syndrome.'   Alcoholism: Clinical and Experimental Research, 3, 195 (abstract).

1649.   SHERWIN, B.T., JACOBSON, S., TROXELL, S.L., ROGERS, A.E., and PELHAM, R.W.   (1980)   'A rat model (using a semipurified diet) of the fetal alcohol syndrome.'   Currents in Alcoholism.   Volume 7: Recent Advances in Research and Treatment.   Ed. M. Galanter.   New York: Grune and Stratton, pp. 15-30.

1650.   SHERWIN, B.T., ZAGORSKI, D., and JACOBSON, S.   (1980)   'Effects of prenatal exposure to ethanol on the development of the rat brain: A model of the fetal alcoholic syndrome.'   Alcoholism: Clinical and Experimental Research, 4, 228 (abstract).

1651. SHERWIN-PHIPPPS, B., and JACOBSON, S. (1981) 'Consequences of
       prenatal ethanol exposure in the rat.' Alcoholism: Clin-
       ical and Experimental Research, 5, 168 (abstract).

1652. SHETTLES, L.B. (1981) 'Ethanol and premature infants.' [Let-
       ter.] American Journal of Obstetrics and Gynecology, 140,
       351.

1653. SHIMMY, Y. (1980) 'Pregnancy and alcoholic drinking.' Josanpu
       Zasshi, 34, 185-190.

1654. SHIN, S.H., and HOWITT, C. (1975) 'Effects of castration on
       luteinizing hormone and luteinizing hormone releasing factor
       in the male rat.' Journal of Endocrinology (London), 65,
       447-448.

1655. SHIOTA, K., CHOU, M.J., and NISHIMURA, H. (1976) 'Factors as-
       sociated with the occurrence of early resorption of human
       embryos.' Mutation Research, 38, 347-348.

1656. SHIOTA, K., and MATSUNAGA, E. (1976) 'Epidemiological study of
       holoprosencephaly in human embryos.' Teratology, 14, 253.

1657. SHOEMAKER, W., BAETGE, G., AZAD, R., SAPIN, V., and BLOOM, F.
       (1981) 'Intrauterine exposure to ethanol: Effect on brain
       neuropeptides and catecholamines.' Teratology, 24, 57A-58A
       (abstract).

1658. SHOEMAKER, W.J., KODA, L.Y., SHOEMAKER, C.A., and BLOOM, F. E.
       (1980) 'Ethanol effects in chick embryos: Cerebellar Pur-
       kinje neurons.' Neurobehavioral Toxicology, 2, 239-242.

1659. SHOEMAKER, W.J., KODA, L.Y., WIENER, S.G., and BLOOM, F.E. (1980)
       'Animal models of fetal alcohol syndrome (FAS): Toxicity
       or teratogenicity.' Teratology, 21, 69A (abstract).

1660. SHOLTY, M.J. (1979) 'Female sexual experience and satisfaction
       as related to alcohol consumption.' Unpublished manuscript.
       Alcohol and Drug Abuse Program, University of Maryland at
       Baltimore.

1661. SHUMAN, R.M., ADICKES, E.D., JACOBSEN, J., and KADER, F.J. (1981)
       'Fetal alcohol myopathy.' Laboratory Investigator, 44,
       7P.

1662. SHURYGIN, G.I. (1974) 'Ob osobennostiiakh psikhicheskogo raz-
       vitiia detei ot materei, stradaiuschikh khronicheskim alko-
       golizmom.' ['Characteristics of the mental development of
       children of alcoholic mothers.'] Pediatriia (Moscow), 11,
       71-73.

1663. SIEGEL, H.I., DOERR, H.K., and ROSENBLATT, J.S. (1978) 'Further
       studies on estrogen-induced maternal behavior in hyster-
       ectomized-ovariectomized virgin rats.' Physiological Behav-
       ior, 21, 99-103.

1664.   SILBER, A., GOTTSCHALK, W., and SARNOFF, C. (1960) 'Alcoholism
        in pregnancy.' Psychiatric Quarterly, 34, 461-471.

1665.   SIMMONDS, H. (1898) 'Über die Ursache der Azoospermie.' ['On
        the cause of inability to produce spermatozoa.'] Inter-
        nationale Monatsschrift, 8, 383.

1666.   SIMMONDS, K. (1898) 'Über die Ursachen der Azoospermie.' ['On
        the causes of inability to produce spermatozoa.'] Berliner
        Klinische Wochenschrift (Berlin), 36, 806.

1667.   SIPPEL, H.W., and KESÄNIEMI, Y.A. (1975) 'Placental and foetal
        metabolism of acetaldehyde in the rat. II. Studies on
        metabolism of acetaldehyde in the isolated placenta and
        foetus.' Acta Pharmacologia et Toxicologica (Copenhagen),
        37, 49-55.

1668.   SITZMANN, F.C. (1980) 'Die Alkohol-Embryofetopathie.' ['Alcohol
        embryofetopathy.'] Zeitschrift für Alternsforschung (Stutt-
        gart), 56, 985-989.

1669.   SJOBLOM, M., OISUND, J.-F., and MORLUND, J. (1979) 'Development
        of alcohol dehydrogenase and aldehyde dehydrogenase in the
        offspring of female rats chronically treated with ethanol.'
        Acta Pharmacologica et Toxicologica (Copenhagen), 44, 128-131.

1670.   SJOBLOM, M., PILSTROM, L., and MORLAND, J. (1978) 'Activity of
        alcohol dehydrogenase and acetaldehyde dehydrogenase in the
        liver and placenta during the development of the rat.'
        Enzyme, 23, 108-115.

1671.   SKAKUN, N.P., VORONTSOV, A.A., SKAKUN, G.K., and SHENDEVITSKIĬ,
        V.I. (1980) 'Alkogol'niĭ sindrom ploda (obzor literaturi).'
        ['Fetal alcohol syndrome: A review of the literature.']
        Voprosy Okhrany Materinstva Detstva, 25, 58-62.

1672.   SKOSYREVA, A.M. (1973) 'Vliyaniye étilovogo spirta na razvitie
        émbrionov stadii organogeneza.' ['The effect of ethyl
        alcohol on the development of embryos at the organogenesis
        stage.'] Akusherstvo i Ginekologiia (Moscow), 4, 15-18.

1673.   SKOSYREVA, A.M. (1977) 'O deistrii alkogolya na potomstvo.'
        ['The effect of alcohol on offspring.'] Akusherstvo i
        Ginekologiia (Moscow), 1, 8-11.

1674.   SKOSYREVA, A.M. (1980) 'Action of ethyl alcohol in the period
        of ontogeny.' Akusherstvo i Ginekologiia (Moscow), 12, 7-9.

1675.   SKOSYREVA, A.M. (1980) 'Deĭstvii alkogolya na plod i potomstvo.'
        ['Action of alcohol on the fetus and progeny.'] Fel'dsher i
        Akusherko, 45, 28-30.

1676.   SKOSYREVA, A.M., BALIKA, I.U.D., and KARTASHEVA, V.E. (1981)
        'Experimental effect of ethyl alcohol on embryonic and
        fetal development.' Akusherstvo i Ginekologiia (Moscow),
        1, 38-40.

1677. SLAVNEY, P.R., and GRAU, J.G.   (1978)   'Fetal alcohol damage and
       schizophrenia.' Journal of Clinical Psychiatry, 39, 782-783.

1678. ŚLEBODZIŃSKI, A.B.   (1979)   'Influence of ethanol on thyroxine
       accumulation in the hypothalamus, pituitary gland and cere-
       brospinal fluid in the newborn rabbit.' Experientia, 35,
       549-550.

1679. SLOTKIN, T.A. and THADANI, P.V.   (1980)   'Neurochemical tera-
       tology of drugs of abuse.' Advanced Study of Birth Defects,
       4, 199-234.

1680. SMALL, W.E.   (1979)   'Warning: Alcohol may be hazardous to your
       baby.' American Pharmacologist, 19, 16-17.

1681. SMITH, D.F.   (1980)   'Intrinsic defects in FAS: Renal, skeletal,
       and cardiac.' Paper presented at the Fetal Alcohol Syndrome
       Workshop, Seattle, Washington (May 2-4).

1682. SMITH, D.F., SANDER, G.G., MACLEOD, P.M., TREDWELL, S., WOOD, B.,
       and NEWMAN, D.E.   (1981)   'Intrinsic defects in the fetal
       alcohol syndrome: Studies on 76 cases from British Columbia
       and the Yukon territory.' Neurobehavioral Toxicology and
       Teratology, 3, 145-152.

1683. SMITH, D.W.   (1977)   'Fetal alcohol syndrome: A tragic and pre-
       ventable disorder.' In: Alcoholism: Development, Conse-
       quences, and Interventions. Ed. N.J. Estes and M.E. Heine-
       mann. St. Louis: The C.V. Mosby Company, pp. 144-149.

1684. SMITH, D.W.   (1978)   'The foetal alcohol syndrome. A tragic and
       preventable disorder.' All Faith's World Alcohol Project
       Journal, 1, 9-15.

1685. SMITH, D.W.   (1979)   'Fetal drug syndromes: Effects of ethanol
       and hydantoins.' Pediatrics in Review, 1, 165-172.

1686. SMITH, D.W.   (1979)   'The fetal alcohol syndrome.' Hospital
       Practice, 14, 121-128.

1687. SMITH, D.W.   (1980)   'Alcohol effects on the fetus.' In: Psycho-
       pharmacology of Alcohol. Ed. Merton Sandler. New York:
       Raven Press, pp. 257-263.

1688. SMITH, D.W.   (1980)   'Alcohol effects on the fetus. In: Pro-
       gress in Clinical and Biological Research. Volume 36: Drug
       and Chemical Risks to the Fetus and Newborn: Proceedings
       of a Symposium. Ed. . Yaffe. New York: Alan R. Liss,
       pp. 73-82.

1689. SMITH, D.W.   (1981)   'Fetal alcohol syndrome and fetal alcohol
       effects.' Neurobehavioral Toxicology and Teratology, 3, 127.

1690.   SMITH, D.W., and GRAHAM, J.M., JR. (1979) 'Reply to "Fetal alco-
hol syndrome in child whose parents had stopped drinking,"
A.P. Scheiner, C.M. Donovan, and L.E. Bartoshevsky.' Lancet
(London), 2, 527.

1691.   SMITH, D.W., JONES, K.L., and HANSON, J.W. (1976) 'Perspectives
on the cause and frequency of the fetal alcohol syndrome.'
Annals of the New York Academy of Sciences, 273, 138-139.

1692.   SMITH, I.E. (1979) 'Fetal alcohol syndrome: A review.' Journal of the Medical Association of Georgia, 68, 799-804.

1693.   SMITH, R.J. (1978) 'Agency drags its feet in warning to pregnant women.' Science, 199, 748-749.

1694.   SMITH, W.H., and HELWIG, F.C. (1940) Liquor: The Servant of
Man. Boston: Little, Brown, and Company.

1695.   SMITHELLS, R.W. (1976) 'Environmental teratogens of man.' British Medical Bulletin, 32, 27-33.

1696.   SMITHELLS, R.W. (1979) 'Fetal alcohol syndrome.' Developmental
Medical and Child Neurology, 21, 244-248.

1697.   SNEED, R.C. (1977) 'The fetal alcohol syndrome. Is alcohol,
lead, or something else the culprit?' [Letter.] Journal of
Pediatrics, 91, 324.

1698.   SNINMI, Y. (1980) 'Pregnancy and alcoholic drinking.' [In
Japanese.] Josanpu Zasshi [Journal for Japanese Midwives],
34, 185-190.

1699.   SOKOL, R.J. (1978) 'Perinatal concomitants of a clinically
recognized alcohol problem during pregnancy: Summary of a
prospective survey.' U.S. Senate, Subcommittee on Alcoholism
and Drug Abuse of the Committee on Human Resources (Wil-
liam D. Hathaway, Chairman). Alcohol Labeling and Fetal
Alcohol Syndrome, The 95th Congress, Second Session, S. 1464,
pp. 164-168.

1700.   SOKOL, R.J. (1980) 'Alcohol abuse during pregnancy: Clinical
research problems.' Teratology, 21, 70A (abstract).

1701.   SOKOL, R.J. (1980) 'Alcohol and spontaneous abortion.' Lancet
(London), 2, 1079.

1702.   SOKOL, R.J. (1980) 'Alcohol-in-pregnancy: Clinical research
problems.' Neurobehavioral Toxicology, 2, 157-165.

1703.   SOKOL, R.J. (1980) 'The Cleveland study.' Paper presented at
the Fetal Alcohol Syndrome Workshop, Seattle, Washington
(May 2-4).

1704.   SOKOL, R.J. (1981) 'Alcohol and abnormal outcomes of pregnancy.'
Canadian Medical Association Journal, 125, 143-148.

1705. SOKOL, R.J., and MILLER, S.I.   (1980)   'Identifying the alcohol-
      abusing obstetric/gynecologic patient: A practical ap-
      proach.' Unpublished report.

1706. SOKOL, R.J., MILLER, S.I., DEBANNE, S., GOLDEN, N., COLLINS, G.,
      KAPLAN, J., and MARTIER, S.   (1981)   'The Cleveland NIAAA
      prospective alcohol-in-pregnancy study: The first year.'
      Neurobehavioral Toxicology and Teratology, 3, 203-209.

1707. SOKOL, R.J., MILLER, S.I., and REED, G.   (1980)   'Alcohol abuse
      during pregnancy: An epidemiologic study.' Alcoholism:
      Clinical and Experimental Research, 4, 135-145.

1708. SOKOL, R.J., STOJKOV, J., and CHIK, L.   (1979)   'Maternal-fetal
      risk assessment: A clinical guide to monitoring.' Clinical
      Obstetrics and Gynecology, 22, 547-560.

1709. SOLLIER, P.   (1889)   'Le role de l'heredité dans l'alcoolisme.'
      ['The role of heredity in alcoholism.'] Thèse, Paris.

1710. SOLOMON, S.   (1977)   'Fetal alcohol syndrome.' Previews, 6, 3.

1711. SONNICHSEN, B.   (1974)   'Innocent victim.' Listen, 27, 14-15.

1712. SORETTE, M.P., MAGGIO, C.A., STARPOLI, A., BOISSEVAIN, A.L., and
      GREENWOOD, M.R.C.   (1980)   'Effect of moderate and high mater-
      nal alcohol intake on fetal development.' Federation Pro-
      ceedings, 39 (abstract #3058).

1713. SORETTE, M.P., MAGGIO, C.A., STARPOLI, A., BOISSEVAIN, A., and
      GREENWOOD, M.R.C.   (1980)   'Maternal ethanol intake affects
      rat organ development despite adequate nutrition.' Neuro-
      behavioral Toxicology, 2, 181-188.

1714. SOUTHREN, A.L,, and GORDON, G.G.   (1976)   'Effects of alcohol and
      alcoholic cirrhosis on sex hormone metabolism.' Fertility
      and Sterility, 27, 202-206.

1715. SOUTHREN, A.L., and GORDON, G.G.   (1970)   'Studies in androgen
      metabolism.' Mount Sinai Journal of Medicine, 37, 516-527.

1716. SOUTHREN, A.L., GORDON, G.G., OLIVO, J., ROSENTHAL, W.S., and
      RAFII, F.   (1973)   'Androgen metabolism in cirrhosis of the
      liver.' Metabolism, 22, 695-702.

1717. SOUTHREN, A.L., GORDON, G.G., and TOCHIMOTO, S.   (1968)   'Further
      study of factors affecting the metabolic clearance rate of
      testosterone in man.' Journal of Clinical Endocrinology and
      Metabolism, 28, 1108-1112.

1718. SPAANS, C., and VERSPREET, F.A.M.   (1981)   'Het foetale alcohol-
      syndroom: Vier patiënten in één gezin.' ['Fetal alcohol
      syndrome: 4 patients in one family.'] Ned Tijdschrift
      Geneeskunde, 125, 452-454.

1719. SPARROW, D., BOSSE, R., and ROWE, J.W. (1980) 'The influence of age, alcohol consumption, and body build on gonadal function in men.' Journal of Clinical Endocrinology and Metabolism, 51, 508-512.

1720. SPEARING, G. (1979) 'Alcohol, indomethacin, and salbutanol: A comparative trial of their use in preterm labor.' Obstetrics and Gynecological Survey, 53, 171-174.

1721. SPIEGAL, P.G., PEKMAN, W.M., RICH, B.H., VERSTEEG, C.N., NELSON, V., and DUDNIKOV, M. (1979) 'The orthopedic aspects of the fetal alcohol syndrome.' Clinica Orthopaedics and Related Research, 139, 58-63.

1722. SPRANGER, J. (1981) 'Attention deficit syndrome in children born to alcoholic mothers.' [Letter.] Journal of Pediatrics, 98, 670.

1723. STAISEY, N., and FRIED, P. (1981) 'Relationships between moderate maternal alcohol consumption during pregnancy and infant neurological development.' Paper presented at the Eastern Psychological Association, New York (April).

1724. STEEG, C.N., and WOOLF, P. (1979) 'Cardiovascular malformations in the fetal alcohol syndrome.' American Heart Journal, 98, 635-637.

1725. STEER, C.M., and PETRIE, R.H. (1977) 'A comparison of magnesium sulfate and alcohol for the prevention of premature labor.' American Journal of Obstetrics and Gynecology, 129, 1-4.

1726. STEKHUN, F.I. (1979) 'Alkogol' i tabakokureniye kak vozmozhnyye prichiny besplodiya muzhchin.' ['Alcohol and tobacco smoking as possible causes of sterility in men.'] Vestnik Dermatologii I Venerologii, 7, 61-65.

1727. STEKHUN, F.I. (1979) 'Vliyaniye alkogolya na muzhskiye polovye zhelezy.' ['Influence of alcohol on the male sexual glands.'] Zhurnal Nevropatologii i Psikhiatrii imeni s s Korsakova (Moscow), 79, 192-195.

1728. STEWART, B. (1979) 'The fetal alcohol syndrome.' The Pharm-Chem Newsletter, 8, 1-4.

1729. STOCKARD, C.R. (1910) 'The influence of alcohol and other anaesthetics on embryonic development.' American Journal of Anatomy, 10, 369-392.

1730. STOCKARD, C.R. (1911) 'The influence of alcohol and other anaesthetics on embryonic development.' Journal of Inebriety, 33, 176-182.

1731. STOCKARD, C.R. (1911-1912) 'The influence of alcoholism on the offspring.' Proceedings of the Society of Experimental Biology and Medicine, 9, 76.

1732.   STOCKARD, C.R.   (1912)   'An experimental study of racial degener-
         ation in mammals treated with alcohol.'   Archives of Inter-
         nal Medicine, 10, 369-398.

1733.   STOCKARD, C.R.   (1913)   'The effect on the offspring of intox-
         icating the male parent and the transmission of the defects
         to the subsequent generations.'   American Naturalist, 47,
         641-682.

1734.   STOCKARD, C.R.   (1913-14)   'The artificial production of struc-
         tural arrests and racial degeneration.'   Proceedings of the
         New York Pathological Society, 13, 83-89.

1735.   STOCKARD, C.R.   (1914)   'A study of further generations of mam-
         mals from ancestors treated with alcohol.'   Proceedings of
         the Society for Experimental Biology and Medicine, 11,
         136-139.

1736.   STOCKARD, C.R.   (1914)   'The artificial production of eye ab-
         normalities in the chick embryo.'   Anatomical Record, 8,
         33-41.

1737.   STOCKARD, C.R.   (1916)   'A study of further generations of mam-
         mals treated with alcohol.'   Proceedings of the Society for
         Expermental Biology and Medicine, 11, 136.

1738.   STOCKARD, C.R.   (1916)   'The heredity transmission of degeneracy
         and deformities by the descendants of alcoholized mammals.'
         Interstate Medical Journal, 23, 385-403.

1739.   STOCKARD, C.R.   (1922)   'Alcohol as a selective agent in the
         improvement of racial stock.'   British Medical Journal
         (London), 2, 255-260.

1740.   STOCKARD, C.R.   (1923)   'Experimental modifications of the germ-
         plasm and its bearing on the inheritance of acquired char-
         acters.'   Proceedings of the American Philosophical Society,
         62, 311-325.

1741.   STOCKARD, C.R.   (1924)   'Alcohol a factor in eliminating racial
         degeneracy.'   American Journal of the Medical Sciences,
         167, 469-477.

1742.   STOCKARD, C.R.   (1932)   'The effects of alcohol in develop-
         ment and heredity.'   In: Alcohol and Man.   Ed. H. Emerson.
         New York: Macmillan, pp. 103-119.

1743.   STOCKARD, C.R., and CRAIG, D.M.   (1912)   'An experimental study
         of the influence of alcohol on the germ cells and the de-
         veloping embryos of mammals.'   Archives für Entwicklungs-
         mechanik der Organismen (Leipzig), 35, 569-597.

1744.   STOCKARD, C.R., and PAPANICOLAOU, G.   (1916)   'A further analysis
         of the hereditary transmission of degeneracy and deformities
         by the descendants of alcoholized mammals.'   American
         Naturalist, 50, 65-88, 144-177.

1745.   STOCKARD, C.R., and PAPANICOLAOU, G.A. (1918) 'Further studies
        on the modification of the germ cells in mammals: The ef-
        fect of alcohol on treated guinea-pigs and their descen-
        dants. Journal of Experimental Zoology, 26, 119-226.

1746.   STOEWSNAD, G.S., and ANDERSON, J.L. (1974) 'Influence on wine
        intake on mouse growth, reproduction and changes in tri-
        glyceride and cholesterol metabolism of offspring.' Journal
        of Food Science, 39, 957-961.

1747.   STREISSGUTH, A.P. (1976) 'Maternal alcoholism and the outcome
        of pregnancy: A review of the fetal alcohol syndrome.' In:
        Alcoholism Problems in Women and Children. Ed. M. Green-
        blatt and M.A. Schuckit. New York: Grune and Stratton,
        pp. 251-274.

1748.   STREISSGUTH, A.P. (1976) 'Psychologic handicaps in children
        with the fetal alcohol syndrome.' Annals of the New York
        Academy of Sciences, 273, 140-145.

1749.   STREISSGUTH, A.P. (1977) 'Maternal drinking and the outcome of
        pregnancy: Implications for child mental health.' Amer-
        ican Journal of Orthopsychiatry, 47, 422-431.

1750.   STREISSGUTH, A.P. (1978) 'Development handicaps in the F.A.S.
        child.' Paper presented at Fetal Alcohol Syndrome Sym-
        posium, Ann Arbor, Michigan.

1751.   STREISSGUTH, A.P. (1978) 'Fetal alcohol syndrome: An epi-
        demiologic perspective.' American Journal of Epidemiology,
        107, 467-478.

1752.   STREISSGUTH, A.P. (1979) 'Fetal alcohol syndrome: Where are
        we in 1978?' Women and Health, 4, 223-237.

1753.   STREISSGUTH, A.P. (1980) 'Alcohol: A behavioral teratogen in
        humans.' Paper presented at the 20th Annual Meeting of the
        Teratology Society, Portsmouth, New Hampshire (June 8-12).

1754.   STREISSGUTH, A.P. (1980) 'Álcool como agente teratogênico:
        A sindrome do alcoolismo fetal.' ['Alcohol as a teratogenic
        agent: The fetal alcohol syndrome.'] Revista da Associacao
        Brasileira de Psiquiatria, 2, 121-130.

1755.   STREISSGUTH, A.P. (1980) 'Female alcoholism: Impacts on women
        and children.' In: Currents in Alcoholism. Volume 7:
        Recent Advances in Research and Treatment. Ed. M. Galanter.
        New York: Grune and Stratton, pp. 429-434.

1756.   STREISSGUTH, A.P. (1980) 'Mental development in children of
        alcoholic mothers.' Proceedings from South Carolina Fetal
        Alcohol Syndrome Workshop. University of South Carolina
        School of Medicine.

1757. STREISSGUTH, A.P.   (1980)   'The Seattle longitudinal study.'
       Paper presented at the Fetal Alcohol Syndrome Workshop,
       Seattle, Washington (May 2-4).

1758. STREISSGUTH, A.P.   (1981)   'Summary and recommendations: Epi-
       demiologic and human studies on alcohol and pregnancy.'
       Neurobehavioral Toxicology and Teratology, 3, 241-242.

1759. STREISSGUTH, A.P., BARR, H.M., MARTIN, D.C., and HERMAN, C.
       (1979)   'Effects of maternal alcohol, nicotine, and caffeine
       use during pregnancy on infant development at eight months.'
       Alcoholism: Clinical and Experimental Research, 3, 197
       (abstract).

1760. STREISSGUTH, A.P., BARR, H., MARTIN, D., and HERMAN, C.   (1979)
       'Effects of maternal alcohol, nicotine and caffeine use
       during pregnancy on infant development at eight months.'
       Paper presented at the biennial meeting of the Society
       for Research in Child Development, San Francisco, California.

1761. STREISSGUTH, A.P., BARR, H.M., MARTIN, D.C., and HERMAN, C.S.
       (1980)   'Effects of maternal alcohol, nicotine and caffeine
       use during pregnancy on infant mental and motor development
       at 8 months.' Alcoholism: Clinical and Experimental Re-
       search, 4, 152-164.

1762. STREISSGUTH, A.P., BARR, H.C., MARTIN, D.C., and WOODELL, S.
       (1978) 'Effects of social drinking on Apgar scores and
       neonatal status.' Alcoholism: Clinical and Experimental
       Research, 2, 215 (abstract).

1763. STREISSGUTH, A.P., HERMAN, C.S., and SMITH, D.W.   (1978)   'In-
       telligence, behavior and dysmorphogenesis in the fetal alco-
       hol syndrome: A report on 20 clinical cases.' Journal of
       Pediatrics, 92, 363-367.

1764. STREISSGUTH, A.P., HERMAN, C.S., and SMITH, D.W.   (1978)   'Sta-
       bility of intelligence in the fetal alcohol syndrome: A
       preliminary report.' Alcoholism: Clinical and Experimental
       Research, 2, 165-170.

1765. STREISSGUTH, A.P., LANDESMAN-DWYER, S., MARTIN, J.C., and SMITH,
       D.W.   (1980) 'Teratogenic effects of alcohol in humans and
       laboratory animals.' Science, 209, 353-361.

1766. STREISSGUTH, A.P., and LITTLE, R.E.   (1980)   'Alcohol-related
       morbidity and mortality in offspring of drinking women:
       Methodological issues and a review of the literature.' In:
       Alcoholism and Epidemiology (in press).

1767. STREISSGUTH, A.P., LITTLE, R.E., HERMAN, C., and WOODELL, B.S.
       (1979) 'IQ in children of recovered alcoholic mothers
       compared with matched controls.' Alcoholism: Clinical and
       Experimental Research, 3, 197 (abstract).

1768. STREISSGUTH, A.P., MARTIN, D.C., and BARR, H.M. (1977) 'Neo-
       natal Brazelton assessment and relationship to maternal
       alcohol use.' Paper presented at the 5th International
       Congress on Birth Defects, International Congress Series,
       No. 426, 62.

1769. STREISSGUTH, A.P., MARTIN, D.C., and BARR, H.M. (1980) 'Moderate
       drinking during pregnancy and offspring effects.' Paper pre-
       sented at a Symposium on the Effects of Moderate Drinking,
       American Medical Association, Winter Scientific Meeting,
       San Antonio, Texas (January 12-15).

1770. STREISSGUTH, A.P., MARTIN, D.C., BARR, H.M., and MARTIN, J.C.
       (1977) 'Alcohol, nicotine and caffeine use in 1529 pregnant
       women.' Paper presented at the Western Psychological
       Association Meeting, Seattle, Washington (April).

1771. STREISSGUTH, A.P., MARTIN, D.C., and BUFFINGTON, V.E. (1976)
       'Test-retest reliability of three scales derived from a
       quantity-frequency-variability assessment of self-reported
       alcohol consumption.' Annals of the New York Academy of
       Sciences, 273, 458-466.

1772. STREISSGUTH, A.P., MARTIN, D.C., and BUFFINGTON, V.E. (1977)
       'Identifying heavy drinkers: A comparison of eight alcohol
       scores obtained on the same sample.' In: Currents in Alco-
       holism. Ed. F.A.S. Seixas. New York: Grune and Stratton,
       pp. 395-420.

1773. STREISSGUTH, A.P., MARTIN, D.C., MARTIN, J.C., and BARR, H.M.
       (1980) 'A longitudinal prospective study on the effects of
       intrauterine alcohol exposure in humans.' In: Longitudinal
       Research in the United States. Ed. S. Mednick and M. Harway
       (in press).

1774. STREISSGUTH, A.P., MARTIN, D.C., MARTIN, J.C., and BARR, H.M.
       (1981) 'The Seattle longitudinal prospective study on alco-
       hol and pregnancy.' Neurobehavioral Toxicology and Tera-
       tology, 3, 223-233.

1775. STREISSGUTH, A.P., MARTIN, J.C., and MARTIN, D.C. (1977) 'Exper-
       imental design considerations and methodological problems in
       the study of the effects of social drinking on the outcome of
       pregnancy.' Paper presented at the NIAAA Fetal Alcohol Syn-
       drome Workshop, San Diego, California.

1776. STREISSGUTH, A.P., MARTIN, J.C., and MARTIN, D.C. (1978) 'Exper-
       imental design considerations and methodological problems in
       the study of the effects of social drinking on the outcome of
       pregnancy.' Alcoholism and Drug Abuse Institute Technical
       Report, #78-01, University of Washington, Seattle, Washing-
       ton.

1777.   STREISSGUTH, A.P., MARTIN, J.C., MARTIN, D.C., and BARR, H.M.
        (1977) 'Alcohol and nicotine ingestion in pregnant women.'
        Paper presented at the Western Psychological Association
        Meetings, Seattle, Washington.

1778.   STREISSGUTH, A.P., and SUTHERLAND, N.L. (1980) 'Alcohol and
        pregnancy. Fetal alcohol syndrome, drinking during pregnan-
        cy, and effects on offspring: A bibliography.' Seattle,
        Washington: University of Washington Alcoholism and Drug
        Abuse Institute Technical Report, #79-04.

1779.   STUCKLIK, J. (1915) 'Über die hereditaren Beziehung zwischen
        Alkoholismus und Epilepsie.' ['On the hereditary relation
        between alcoholism and epilepsy.'] Correspondenzblatt für
        Schweizer Ärzte (Basel), 45, 70-84.

1780.   STULL, R.E., PASLEY, J.N., RIDDELL, E.A., and LIGHT, K.E. (1980)
        'Effects of ethanol on brain zinc concentration in mice.'
        Substance Alcohol Actions and Misuse, 1, 565-568.

1781.   STURDEVANT, R. (1974) 'Offspring of chronic alcoholic women.'
        [Letter.] Lancet (London), 2, 349.

1782.   STURGE, M.D., and HORSLEY, V. (1911) 'On some of the biological
        and statistical errors in the work on parental alcoholism by
        Miss Elderton and Professor Karl Pearson.' British Medical
        Journal (London), 1, 72-83.

1783.   SULIK, K.K., JOHNSTON, M.C., and WEBB, M.A. (1981) "Fetal alco-
        hol syndrome: Embryogenesis on a mouse model.' Science,
        214, 936-938.

1784.   SULLIVAN, W.C. (1899) 'A note on the influence of maternal in-
        ebriety on the offspring.' Journal of Mental Science (Lon-
        don), 45, 489-503.

1785.   SULLIVAN, W.C. (1899) 'Influence of maternal inebriety on the
        offspring.' Glasgow Medical Journal (Glasgow), 52, 292.

1786.   SULLIVAN, W.C. (1900) 'The children of the female drunkard.'
        Medical Temperance Review, 3, 72-79.

1787.   SULLIVAN, W.C. (1906) Alcoholism and Degeneration. London.

1788.   SUMMERSKILL, W.H.J., DAVIDSON, C.S., DIBLE, J.H., MALLORY, G.K.,
        SHERLOCK, S., TURNER, M.D., and WOLFE, S.J. (1960) 'Cir-
        rhosis of the liver: A study of alcoholic and nonalcoholic
        patients in Boston and London.' New England Journal of
        Medicine, 262, 1-9.

1789.   SUZUKI, A., MORITA, C., and NAKAMURA, K. (1967) 'A study on
        morphological changes of the rat brain transplacentally
        treated with ethanol prenatally.' Proceedings of the
        Congenital Anomalies Research Associates Annual Report
        (Japan), 7, 65.

1790.   SUZUKI, N., TANAKA, H., and ARIMA, M.   (1980)   'Fetal and post-
        natal biochemical development in the fetal alcohol syndrome
        of the rats.'   [In Japanese.]   No To Shinkei [Brain and
        Nerve] (Tokyo), 32, 1136-1142 (abstract).

1791.   SWANBERG, K.M.   (1977)   'Relationships between adrenal cortico-
        steroids and alcohol tolerance: The effects of neonatal ex-
        posure to alcohol on mice selectively bred for different
        sensitivities to alcohol.'   Dissertation Abstracts Inter-
        national, 37, (12-13, Part 2), 6397 (abstract).

1792.   SWANBERG, K.M., and CRUMPACKER, D.W.   (1977)   'Genetic differ-
        ences in reproductive fitness and offspring viability in
        mice exposed to alcohol during gestation.'   Behavioral Bio-
        logy, 20, 122-127.

1793.   SWANBERG, K.M., and WILSON, J.R.   (1979)   'Genetic and ethanol-
        related differences in maternal behavior and offspring via-
        bility in mice.'   Developmental Psychobiology, 12, 61-66.

1794.   SWANBERG, K.M., WILSON, J.R., and KALISKER, A.   (1979)   'Develop-
        mental and genotypic effects on pituitary-adrenal function
        and alcohol tolerance in mice.'   Developmental Psychobio-
        logy, 12, 201-210.

1795.   SYMONS, A.M., and MARKS, V.   (1975)   'The effects of alcohol on
        weight gain and the hypothalamic-pituitary-gonadotrophin
        axis in the maturing male rat.'   Biochemical Pharmacology,
        24, 955-958.

1796.   SZE, P.Y., YANAI, J., and GINSBURG, B.E.   (1976)   'Effects of
        early ethanol input on the activities of ethanol-metabolizing
        enzymes in mice.'   Biochemical Pharmacology, 25, 215-217.

1797.   SZOKE, M.C., MALONE, M.J., and ROSMAN, N.P.   (1977)   'Effect of
        ethanol on the developing nervous system.'   Transactions
        of the American Society of Neurochemistry, 6, 231.

T

1798. TABAKOFF, B. (1981) 'Summary and recommendations for biochemical studies of the fetal alcohol syndrome.' Neurobehavioral Toxicology and Teratology, 3, 235.

1799. TABAKOFF, B., NOBLE, E.P., and WARREN, K.R. (1979) 'Alcohol nutrition and the brain.' In: Nutrition and the Brain. Volume 4: Toxic Effects of Food Constituents on the Brain. Ed. R.J. Wurtman and J.J. Wurtman. New York: Raven Press, pp. 159-214.

1800. TAMERIN, J.S., WEINER, S., and MENDELSON, J.H. (1970) 'Alcoholics' expectancies and recall of experiences during intoxication.' American Journal of Psychiatry, 126, 39-46.

1801. TANAKA, H., and ARIMA, M. (1979) 'Effects of maternal alcohol consumption on fetal, perinatal and postnatal development in the rat.' Teratology, 20, 156 (abstract).

1802. TANAKA, H., SUZUKI, N., and ARIMA, M. (1980) 'Hypoglycemia in the fetal alcohol syndrome in rats.' Teratology, 22, 20A (abstract).

1803. TANAKA, H., SUZUKI, N., and ARIMA, M. (1980) 'The fetal alcohol syndrome in rats.' Igaku No Ayumi, 115, 929-932.

1804. TARACHAND, U., and EAPEN, J. (1977) 'Effect of ethanol on placenta and liver of mice.' Indian Journal of Experimental Biology (New Delhi), 15, 274-276.

1805. TARTER, R.E. (1980) 'Menstrual distress and its relationship to experienced craving, personality and sex role conflict.' Alcoholism: Clinical and Experimental Research, 4, 230 (abstract).

1806. TATES, A.D., DE-VOGEL, N., and NEUTEBOOM, I. (1980) 'Cytogenetic effects in hepatocytes, bone-marrow cells and blood lymphocytes of rats exposed to ethanol in the drinking water.' Mutation Research (Amsterdam), 79, 285-288.

1807.   TATES, A.D., and NATARAJAN, A.T.   (1976) 'A correlative study on
           the genetic damage induced by chemical mutagens in bone mar-
           row and spermatogonia of mice. I. CNU-ethanol.' Mutation
           Research (Amsterdam), 37, 267-277.

1808.   TAYLOR, A.N., BRANCH, B.J., LIU, S., and KOKKA, N. (1980) 'Fetal
           exposure to alcohol enhances pituitary-adrenal and hypother-
           mic responses to alcohol in adult rats.' Alcoholism: Clin-
           ical and Experimental Research, 4, 231 (abstract).

1809.   TAYLOR, A.N., BRANCH, B.J., LIU, S.H., and KOKKA, N. (1981) 'Evi-
           dence for enhanced pituitary-adrenal and behavioral responses
           to stress in adult rats exposed to alcohol in utero.' Alco-
           holism: Clinical and Experimental Research, 5, 169 (ab-
           stract).

1810.   TAYLOR, A.N., BRANCH, B.J., LIU, S.H., WEICHMANN, A.F., HILL,
           M.A., and KOKKA, N. (1981) 'Fetal exposure to ethanol en-
           hances pituitary-adrenal and temperature responses to eth-
           anol in adult rats.' Alcoholism: Clinical and Experimental
           Research, 5, 237-246.

1811.   TAYLOR, A.N., LIU, S.H., RANDOLPH, D., BRANCH, B.J., and KOKKA, N.
           (1981) 'Fetal exposure to ethanol alters drug sensitivity in
           adult rats.' Alcoholism: Clinical and Experimental Re-
           search, 5, 169 (abstract).

1812.   TEITELBAUM, H.A., and GANTT, W.H. (1958) 'The effect of alcohol
           on sexual reflexes and sperm count in the dog.' Quarterly
           Journal of Studies on Alcohol, 19, 394-398.

1813.   TENBRINCK, M.S., and BUCHIN, S.Y. (1975) 'Fetal alcohol syn-
           drome: Report of a case.' Journal of the American Medical
           Association, 232, 1144-1147.

1814.   TENNES, K., and BLACKARD, C. (1980) 'Maternal alcohol consump-
           tion, birth weight, and minor physical anomalies.' American
           Journal of Obstetrics and Gynecology, 138, 774-780.

1815.   TEPPERMAN, H.M., BEYDOUN, S.N., and ABDUL-KARIM, R.W.   (1977)
           'Drugs affecting myometrial contractility in pregnancy.'
           Clinical Obstetrics and Gynecology, 20, 423-445.

1816.   TERNISIEN, J., and VANHOOVE, D. (1977) 'Les cardiopathies des
           enfants nés de mère alcoolique chronique. À propos de
           42 observations.' ['The cardiopathies of infants born to
           chronically alcoholic mothers. Regarding 42 observations.']
           Thèse de médicine, Lille.

1817.   TERRAPON, M., SCHNEIDER, P., FRIEDLI, B., and COX, J.N. (1977)
           'Aortic arch interruption type A with aortopulmonary
           fenestration in an offspring of a chronic alcoholic mother
           ("fetal alcohol syndrome").' Helvetica Paediatrica Acta
           (Basel), 32, 141-148.

1818.   TESCHER, M. RUDELIN, D., and MALOUX, G.   (1978)   'Drogues et tabac
        pendant la grossesse.'   ['Drugs and tobacco in pregnancy.']
        Revue Pratique, 28, 809-812, 815-816, 819.

1819.   THADANI, P.V.   (1980)   'Effect of a single dose of ethanol admin-
        istered to pregnant rats on developing brain and heart orni-
        thine decarboxylase activity.'   Federation Proceedings, 39
        (abstract #463).

1820.   THADANI, P.V.   (1981)   'Effect of maternal ethanol ingestion on
        development of sympathetic neurotransmission in heart of
        developing rats.'   Alcoholism: Clinical and Experimental
        Research, 5, 170 (abstract).

1821.   THADANI, P.V., LAU, C., SLOTKIN, T.A., and SCHANBERG, S.M.
        (1977)   'Effects of maternal ethanol ingestion on amine up-
        take into synaptosomes of fetal and neonatal rat brain.'
        Journal of Pharmacology and Experimental Therapeutics, 200,
        292-297.

1822.   THADANI, P.V., LAU, C., SLOTKIN, T.A., and SCHANBERG, S.M.   (1977)
        'Effects of maternal ethanol ingestion on neonatal rat brain
        and heart ornithine decarboxylase.'   Biochemical Pharmacol-
        ogy, 26, 523-527.

1823.   THADANI, P.V., and SCHANBERG, S.M.   (1979)   'Effect of maternal
        ethanol ingestion on serum growth hormone in the developing
        rat.'   Neuropharmacology (Oxford), 18, 821-826.

1824.   THADANI, P.V., SLOTKIN, T.A., and SCHANBERG, S.M.   (1977)   'Ef-
        fects of late prenatal or early postnatal ethanol exposure
        on ornithine decarboxylase activity in brain and heart of
        developing rats.'   Neuropharmacology (Oxford), 16, 289-293.

1825.   THANASSI, N.M., ROKOWSKI, R.J., SHEEHY, J., HART, B., ABSHER, M.,
        and CUTRONEO, K.R.   (1980)   'Non-selective decrease of col-
        lagen synthesis by cultured fetal lung fibroblasts after
        non-lethal doses of ethanol.'   Biochemical Pharmacology, 29,
        2417-2424.

1826.   THE JOURNAL (Toronto).   (1975)   'Jury still out on pregnant
        drinkers.'   December 1, p. 7.

1827.   THE JOURNAL (Toronto).   (1975)   'Women shun the bottle during
        pregnancy: Study.'   February 1, p. 5.

1828.   THE JOURNAL (Toronto).   (1975)   'Birth pill, abortion urged for
        female alcoholics.'   October 1, p. 1.

1829.   THE JOURNAL (Toronto).   (1977)   'Fingerprints for F.A.S.'
        March 1, p. 4.

1830.   THE JOURNAL (Toronto).   (1977)   'Mother's daily beer boosts risk
        of still born.'   March 1, p. 1.

1831. THE JOURNAL (Toronto). (1979) 'An "alcoholic binge" helped in her delivery.' July 1, page 7.

1832. THE JOURNAL (Toronto). (1979) 'FAS parents should sue.' Volume 8, p. 2.

1833. THE JOURNAL (Toronto). (1980) 'What they're saying about FAS.' Volume 9, p. 9.

1834. THEMA ZUM PACHE, H.-D. (1976) 'Alkohol-Embryopathie.' ['Alcohol embryopathology.'] Münchener Medizinische Wochenschrift (Munich), 118, 7-8.

1835. THIEME, G., and NEUMANN, J. (1980) 'Alkoholembryopathie.' ['Alcohol embryopathy.'] Psychiatrie, Neurologie und Medizinische Psychologie (Leipzig), 32, 129-139.

1836. THIERSCH, J.B. (1971) 'Investigations into the differential effect of compounds on rat litter and mother.' In: Congenital Malformations of Mammals.   Paris: Masson and Cie, pp. 95-113.

1837. THIESSEN, D.D., WHITWORTH, N.S., and RODGERS, D.A. (1966) 'Reproductive variables and alcohol consumption of the C57BL/Crgl female mouse.' Quarterly Journal of Studies on Alcohol, 27, 591-595.

1838. THOMPSON, M.A. (1980) 'Alcohol and pregnancy--Part 2: Studies in man.' Food and Cosmetic Toxicology, 18, 314-316.

1839. THOMPSON, P.A., and FOLB, P.I. (1980) 'Evaluation of central nervous system toxicity in the fetal alcohol syndrome in experimental mice.' Toxicology Letters (Special Issue 1), Second International Congress on Toxicology, Brussels, Belgium (July 6-11), p. 108.

1840. THOMPSON, R.J., JR. (1979) 'Effects of maternal alcohol consumption on offspring: Review, critical assessment, and future directions.' Journal of Pediatric Psychology, 4, 265-276.

1841. TICHÁ, R. (1979) 'Alkoholismus matky jako příčina defektnosti dítěte.' ['Maternal alcoholism as the cause of defects in children.'] Protialkoholi Obzor (Bratislava), 14, 129-132.

1842. TICHÁ, R. (1979) 'Alkoholová embryopatie.' ['Alcohol embryopathy.'] Československa Gynekologie (Prague), 34, 615-617.

1843. TICHÁ, R. (1979) 'Poškození plodu chronickým alkoholismem matky.' ['Fetal damage caused by chronic maternal alcoholism.'] Československa Gynekologie, 44, 341-344.

1844. TILLNER, I., and MAJEWSKI, F. (1978) 'Furrows and dermal ridges of the hand in patients with alcohol embryopathy.' Humangenetik (Berlin), 42, 307-314.

1845. TIME MAGAZINE. (1975) 'Liquor and babies.' July 14, p. 36.

1846. TITTMAR, H.-G. (1973) 'Some effects of alcohol, present during
         the prenatal period, on the development and behavior of
         rats.' Ph.D. Thesis, Queens University, Belfast.

1847. TITTMAR, H.-G. (1974) 'Alcohol intoxication: A method for
         obtaining increased ethanol intake in gravid rats.'
         Journal of Obstetrics and Gynecology, 2, 1079.

1848. TITTMAR, H.-G. (1977) 'Some effects of ethanol, presented
         during the prenatal period, on the development of rats.'
         British Journal on Alcohol and Alcoholism, 12, 71-83.

1849. TITTMAR, H.-G. (1978) 'Some effects of alcohol on reproduction.'
         British Journal on Alcohol and Alcoholism, 13, 122-138.

1850. TITTMAR, H.-G. (1978) 'Some effects of alcohol, presented
         during the prenatal period, on the development and behaviour
         of rats.' Paper presented at the Fourth International Con-
         ference on Alcohol and Drug Abuse, Liverpool.

1851. TO, A., BOYO-EKWUEME, H.T., POSNANSKY, M.C., and LEMAN, D.V.
         (1981) 'Chromosomal abnormalities in ascitic fluid from
         patients with alcoholic cirrhosis.' British Medical Journal
         (London), 282, 1659-1660.

1852. TOPIAR, A., and VILC, M. (1980) 'Zoofilní aktivity v alko-
         holickém opojení.' ['Zoophilic activities during alcohol
         intoxication.'] Protialkoholický Obzor (Bratislava), 15,
         33-35.

1853. TORO, G., KOLODNY, R.C., JACOBS, L.S., MASTERS, W.H., and
         DAUGHADAY, W.H. (1973) 'Failure of alcohol to alter pitui-
         tary and target organ hormone levels.' Clinical Research,
         21, 505 (abstract).

1854. TOUTANT, C., and LIPPMANN, S. (1979) 'Fetal solvents syndrome.'
         [Letter.] Lancet (London), 1, 1356.

1855. TOUTANT, C., and LIPPMANN, S. (1980) 'Fetal alcohol syndrome.'
         American Family Physician, 21, 113-117.

1856. TREDGOLD, A.F. (1908) Mental Deficiency. London.

1857. TREDGOLD, A.F. (1908) Mental Deficiency (Amentia). New York,
         p. 409.

1858. TREDGOLD, A.F. (1909) 'Clinical lecture on feebleminded chil-
         dren.' Medical Press and Circular (London), New Series,
         88, 188-214.

1859. TREDGOLD, A.F. (1909) 'Communication on Dr. W.A. Potts' paper
         on the relation of alcohol to feeblemindedness.' [Letter.]
         British Journal of Inebriety, 6, 146, 156-157.

1860. TROTTER, T. (1813) An Essay, Medical, Philosophical, and Chemical, on Drunkenness, and its Effects on the Human Body. Boston: Bradford and Read.

1861. TROXELL, S., JACOBSON, S., SEHGAL, P., and BURNAP, J. (1981) 'Decreased fertility as a consequence of chronic ethanol consumption in the monkey.' Alcoholism: Clinical and Experimental Research, 5, 170 (abstract).

1862. TUCHMANN-DUPLESSIS, H. (1980) 'Retentissement de l'alcoolisme maternel sur la descendance.' ['Effect on maternal alcoholism in offspring.'] Bulletin de l'Académie Nationale de Médicine, 164, 129-133.

1863. TUCKER, B. (1975) 'Pregnancy and drugs.' Addictions (Toronto), 22, 2-19.

1864. TUMBLESON, M.E. (1977) 'FAS in Sinclair (S-1) miniature swine.' Paper presented at the NIAAA Fetal Alcohol Syndrome Workshop, San Diego, California.

1865. TUMBLESON, M.E., and DEXTER, J.D. (1980) 'Ethanol consumption of gilts farrowed by alcoholic and control miniature swine.' Alcoholism: Clinical and Experimental Research, 4, 231 (abstract).

1866. TURNER, G. (1978) 'The fetal alcohol syndrome.' [Editorial.] Medical Journal of Australia (Sydney), 1, 18-19.

1867. TZE, W.J., FRIESEN, H.G., and MAC LEOD, P.M. (1976) 'Growth hormone response in fetal alcohol syndrome.' Archives of Disease in Childhood (London), 51, 703-706.

1868. TZE, W.J., and LEE, M. (1975) 'Adverse effects of maternal alcohol consumption on pregnancy and foetal growth in rats.' Nature (London), 257, 479-480.

U

1869. UHLIG, H.   (1957) 'Missbildungen unerwünschter Kinder.' ['Mal-
        formations of unwished for children.'] Ärztliche Wochen-
        schrift, 12, 61-65.

1870. ULLELAND, C.N.   (1972) 'The offspring of alcoholic mothers.'
        Annals of the New York Academy of Sciences, 197, 167-169.

1871. ULLELAND, C.N., WENNBERG, R.P., IGO, R.P., and SMITH, N.J.
        (1970) 'The offspring of alcoholic mothers.' Pediatric
        Research, 4, 474 (abstract).

1872. ULLRICH, K.-H., and DIETZMANN, K.   (1980) 'A contribution to
        the postnatal enzymatic state of maturity of gyrus hippo-
        campi in the embryofetal alcohol syndrome of the rat.' Ex-
        perimental Pathology (Jena), 18, 170-174.

1873. UMBREIT, J., and OSTROW, L.S.   (1980) 'The fetal alcohol syn-
        drome.' Mental Retardation, 18, 109-111.

1874. U.S. BUREAU OF ALCOHOL, TOBACCO, AND FIREARMS.   (1978) 'Warning
        labels on containers of alcoholic beverages.' Federal Reg-
        ister, 43, 2186-2187.

1875. U.S. DEPARTMENT OF HEALTH, EDUCATION, AND WELFARE.   (1976; rpt.
        1979) 'De Mujer a Mujer: Hablemos Sobre el Alcoholismo.'
        ['From Woman to Woman: A Conversation on Alcoholism.']
        DHEW Publication No. (ADM) 79-324, 1-9 [brochure].

1876. U.S. DEPARTMENT OF HEALTH, EDUCATION, AND WELFARE.   (1977)
        'Health Caution on Fetal Alcohol Syndrome.' June.

1877. U.S. DEPARTMENT OF HEALTH, EDUCATION, AND WELFARE.   (1978)
        Alcohol and Your Unborn Baby. National Institute on Alcohol
        Abuse and Alcoholism. DHEW Publication No. (ADM) 78-521.

1878. U.S. DEPARTMENT OF HEALTH, EDUCATION, AND WELFARE.   (1980) 'The
        fetal alcohol syndrome.' In: Alcoholism: Introduction to
        Theory and Treatment. Ed. D.A. Ward. Dubuque, Iowa: Ken-
        dall/Hunt, pp. 70-77.

1879. U.S. JOURNAL. (1977) 'Don't drink, pregnant mothers warned.'
        1 (July), p. 3.

1880. U.S. JOURNAL. (1977) 'Fervent support for FAS concerns.'
        2 (December), p. 7.

1881. U.S. JOURNAL. (1977) 'Model program developed to combat FAS.'
        2 (December), p. 7.

1882. U.S. JOURNAL OF DRUG AND ALCOHOL DEPENDENCE. (1979) 'March of
        Dimes warns of FAS.' November 3, p. 15.

V

1883. VALJIN, V., PADELIN, S., and PEROVIĆ, S. (1979) 'Fetalni alko-
       holni sindrom.' ['A case of fetal alcoholic syndrome.']
       Liječnicki Vjesn., 101, 789-791.

1884. VAN BIERVLIET, J.P. (1977) 'The fetal alcohol syndrome.' Acta
       Paediatrie Belge, 30, 113-116.

1885. VAN DEN BERG, B.J. (1977) 'Epidemiologic observations of pre-
       maturity: Effects of behavior, coffee, and alcohol.'
       In: The Epidemiology of Prematurity. Ed. D.M. Reed and
       F.J. Stanley. Baltimore: Urban and Schwarzenberg, pp. 157-
       176.

1886. VAN RENSBURG, L.J. (1981) 'Major skeletal defects in the fetal
       alcohol syndrome: A case report.' South African Medical
       Journal, 59, 687-688.

1887. VAN THIEL, D.H. (1979) 'Feminization of chronic alcoholic men:
       A formulation.' Yale Journal of Biology and Medicine, 52,
       219-225.

1888. VAN THIEL, D.H. (1981) 'Ethanol and pituitary gonadal hormones.'
       Alcoholism: Clinical and Experimental Research, 5, 577-578.

1889. VAN THIEL, D.H., GAVALER, J.S., COBB, C.F., SHERINS, R.J., and
       LESTER, R. (1979) 'Alcohol-induced testicular atrophy in
       the adult male rat.' Endocrinology, 105, 888-895.

1890. VAN THIEL, D.H., GAVALER, J.S., EAGON, P.K., CHIAO, Y.-B., COBB,
       C.F., and LESTER, R. (1980) 'Alcohol and sexual function.'
       Pharmacology, Biochemistry, and Behavior, 13, Supplement 1,
       125-129.

1891. VAN THIEL, D.H., GAVALER, J.S., and LESTER, R. (1974) 'Ethanol
       inhibition of vitamin A metabolism in the testes: Possible
       mechanism for sterility in alcoholics.' Science, 186, 941-
       942.

1892. VAN THIEL, D.H., GAVALER, J.S., and LESTER, R. (1977) 'Ethanol: A gonadal toxin in the female.' Drug and Alcohol Dependence (Lausanne), 2, 373-380.

1893. VAN THIEL, D.H., GAVALER, J.S., and LESTER, R. (1978) 'Alcohol-induced ovarian failure in the rat.' Journal of Clinical Investigation, 61, 624-632.

1894. VAN THIEL, D.H., GAVALER, J.S., LESTER, R., and GOODMAN, M.D. (1975) 'Alcohol-induced testicular atrophy: An experimental model for hypogonadism occurring in chronic alcoholic men.' Gastroenterology, 69, 326-332.

1895. VAN THIEL, D.H., GAVALER, J.S., LESTER, R., LORIAUX, D.L., and BRAUNSTEIN, G.D. (1975) 'Plasma estrone, prolactin, neurophysin, and sex steroid-binding globulin in chronic alcoholic men.' Metabolism: Clinical and Experimental, 24, 1015-1019.

1896. VAN THIEL, D.H., GAVALER, J.S., LESTER, R., and SHERINS, R.J. (1978) 'Alcohol-induced ovarian failure in the rat.' Journal of Clinical Investigation, 61, 624-632.

1897. VAN THIEL, D.H., GAVALER, J.S., SLONE, F.L., COBB, C.F., SMITH, W.I., JR., BRON, K.M., and LESTER, R. (1980) 'Is feminization in alcoholic men due in part to portal hypertension: A rat model." Gastroenterology, 78, 81-91.

1898. VAN THIEL, D.H., and LESTER, R. (1974) 'Sex and alcohol.' New England Journal of Medicine, 291, 251-253.

1899. VAN THIEL, D.H., and LESTER, R. (1976) 'Alcoholism: Its effect on hypothalamic-pituitary-gonadal function.' Gastroenterology, 71, 318-327.

1900. VAN THIEL, D.H., and LESTER, R. (1976) 'Sex and alcohol: A second peek.' New England Journal of Medicine, 295, 826-835.

1901. VAN THIEL, D.H., and LESTER, R. (1979) 'The effect of chronic alcohol abuse on sexual function.' Clinics in Endocrinology and Metabolism, 8, 499-510.

1902. VAN THIEL, D.H., LESTER, R., and SHERINS, R.J. (1974) 'Hypogonadism in alcoholic liver disease: Evidence for a double defect.' Gastroenterology, 67, 1188-1199.

1903. VAN THIEL, D.H., LESTER, R., and VAITUKAITIS, J. (1978) 'Evidence for a defect in pituitary secretion of luteinizing hormone in chronic alcoholic men.' Journal of Clinical Endocrinology and Metabolism, 47, 499-507.

1904. VAN THIEL, D.H., and LORIAUX, D.L. (1979) 'Evidence for an adrenal origin of plasma estrogens in alcoholic men.' Metabolism: Clinical and Experimental, 28, 536-541.

1905.   VAN THIEL, D.H., MC CLAIN, C.J., ELSON, M.K., MC MILLAN, M.J., and
        LESTER, R.   (1978)   'Evidence for autonomous secretion of
        prolactin in some alcoholic men with cirrhosis and gyneco-
        mastia.'   Metabolism: Clinical and Experimental, 27, 1778-
        1784.

1906.   VARGAS OJEDA, A.C., HERMAN, J., MARTINEZ CERON, M.C., RAMIREZ, S.,
        and GONZALEZ-RAMAS, M.   (1976)   'Review of 5 cases of fetal
        alcohol syndrome.'   Excerpta Medica, International Congress
        Series, 397, 105.

1907.   VARMA, P.K., and PERSAUD, T.V.N.   (1979)   'Influence of pyrazole,
        an inhibitor of alcohol dehydrogenase on the prenatal tox-
        icity of ethanol in the rat.'   Research Communications in
        Chemical Pathology and Pharmacology, 26, 65-73.

1908.   VAUGHN, J.S.   (1979)   'The effect of information and influence on
        health beliefs regarding the fetal alcohol syndrome of preg-
        nant women receiving prenatal care in a medical care center.'
        Ph.D. Dissertation, University of Pittsburgh.

1909.   VÉGHELYI, P.V., and LEISZTNER, L.   (1981)   'Fetal alcohol syn-
        drome.'   Akusherstvo i Ginekologiia (Moscow), 1, 36-37.

1910.   VÉGHELYI, P.V., LEISZTNER, L., OSZTOVICS, M., KORÁNYI, G., KARDOS,
        G., and ULLRICH, E.   (1980)   'A foetalis alkohol syndroma
        keletkezése.'   ['Development of the fetal alcohol syndrome.']
        Orvosi Hetilap, 121, 133-135.

1911.   VÉGHELYI, P.V., and OSZTOVICS, M.   (1978)   'The alcohol syndromes:
        The intrarecombigenic effect of acetaldehyde.'   Experientia
        (Basel), 34, 195-196.

1912.   VÉGHELYI, P.V., and OSZTOVICS, M.   (1979)   'Fetal alcohol syndrome
        in child whose parents had stopped drinking.'   Lancet (Lon-
        don), 2, 35-36.

1913.   VÉGHELYI, P.V., OSZTOVICS, M., KARDOS, G., LEISZTNER, L., SZAS-
        ZOVSKY, E., IGALI, S., and IMREI, J.   (1978)   'The fetal
        alcohol syndrome: Symptoms and pathogenesis.'   Acta Paed-
        iatrica Academiae Scientiarum Hungricae (Budapest), 19,
        171-189.

1914.   VÉGHELYI, P.V., OSZTOVICS, M., and SZASZOVSKY, E.   (1978)   'Mater-
        nal alcohol consumption and birth weight.'   [Letter.]   Brit-
        ish Medical Journal (London), 2, 1365-1366.

1915.   VEYLON, R.   (1980)   'La consommation d'alcool au cours de la gros-
        sesse.'   ['The consumption of alcohol during pregnancy.'
        Nouvelle Presse Médicale (Paris), 9, 2521.

1916.   VICTOR, M., and LAURENG, R.   (1978)   'Neurologic complications of
        alcohol abuse: Epidemiologic aspects.'   Advances in Neur-
        ology, 19, 603-617.

1917. VIDWAN, K.S., and MANGURTEN, H.H.   (1977) 'Fetal alcohol syn-
          drome.' Quarterly Pediatric Bulletin, 3, 17-21.

1918. VIGNES, H.   (1941) 'L'intoxication alcoolique et ses effets sur
          la race.' ['Alcoholic intoxication and its effects on race.']
          Revue Anthropologique, 52, 33-42.

1919. VILLERMAULAZ, A.   (1977) 'Syndrome de l'alcoolisme foetal.'
          ['Fetal alcohol syndrome.'] Revue Medicale de la Suisse
          Romande (Lausanne), 97, 613-619.

1920. VINCENT, N.M.   (1958) 'The effects of prenatal alcoholism upon
          motivation, emotionality, and learning in the rat.' Amer-
          ican Psychologist, 13, 401.

1921. VOGEL, I.   (1919) 'Über den Einfluss chronischen Narkotika-
          gebrauchs auf die Funktionen der weiblichen Genitalien.'
          ['On the effect of chronic drug use on female genital func-
          tions.'] Archiv für Frauenkunde und Konstitutionsforschung
          (Wurzburg), 15, 157-163.

1922. VOLK, B.   (1977) 'Verzögerte Kleinhirnentwicklung im Rahmen
          des "Embryofetalen Alkoholsyndroms." Lichtoptische Unter-
          suchungen am Kleinhirn der Ratte.' ['Delayed cerebellar
          histogenesis in "embryofetal alcohol syndrome." Light-
          microscopic investigations in the cerebellum of the rat.']
          Acta Neuropathologica (Berlin), 39, 157-163.

1923. VOLK, B., MALETZ, J., TIEDEMANN, M., MALL, G., KLEIN, C., and
          BERLET, H.H.   (1981) 'Impaired maturation of Purkinje cells
          in the fetal alcohol syndrome of the rat: Light and electron
          microscopic investigations.' Acta Neuropathologica (Berlin),
          54, 19-29.

1924. VOLK, B., MALETZ, J., TIEDEMANN, M., MALL, G., KLEIN, C., and
          BERLET, H.H.   (1981) 'Impaired maturation of Purkinje cells
          in the fetal alcohol syndrome of the rat: Light Microscopic
          and electron microscopic investigations.' Acta Morphologica
          Neerl-Scand., 19, 21-34.

1925. VON-CRIEGERN, T.   (1979) 'Rauchen und Alkoholkonsum in der
          Schwangerschaft: Eine subtile Form der Kindesmisshandlung.'
          ['Smoking and alcohol consumption in pregnancy: A subtle
          form of child abuse.'] Schwestern Revue, 17, 19-20.

1926. VYARE, C.Y., LAANE, and CAARMA, T.M.   (1975) 'Ob izmeneniya
          kracnoi krovi i vneshnego dychaniya pri alkogolisme.' ['
                              .'] Jurnal Nevropatologii i Psik-
          hiatrii Imeni S.S. Korsakova, 75, 250-256.

W

1927. WAGNER, G., and FUCHS, A.R. (1968) 'Effect of ethanol on uterine activity during suckling in post-partum women.' Acta Endocrinologica (Copenhagen), 58, 133-141.

1928. WAGNER, L., WAGNER, G., and GUERRERO, J. (1970) 'Effect of alcohol on premature newborn infants.' American Journal of Obstetrics and Gynecology, 108, 308-315.

1929. WAKHALOO, R.L. (1970) 'Ethyl alcohol drip in threatened premature labour.' Journal of Obstetrics and Gynecology of India, 26, 728-734.

1930. WALKER, N.E. (1967) 'Distribution of chemicals injected into fertile eggs and its effect upon apparent toxicity.' Toxicology and Applied Pharmacology, 10, 290-299.

1931. WALL, J.H. (1937) 'A study of alcoholism in women.' American Journal of Psychiatry, 93, 943.

1932. WALPOLE, I.R., and HOCKEY, A. (1980) 'Fetal alcohol syndrome: Implications to family and society in Australia.' Australia Paediatric Journal, 16, 101-105.

1933. WALSH, A.C. (1977) 'Damaged babies of alcoholic mothers: A rational explanation of the cause of the defects.' Lex et Scientia, 93, 206-209.

1934. WALTERS, J. (1975) 'Birth defects and adolescent pregnancies.' Journal of Home Economics, 67, 23-27.

1935. WALTMAN, R., BONURA, F., NIGRIN, G., and PITAT, C. (1969) 'Ethanol in prevention of hyperbilirubinemia in the newborn: A controlled trial.' Lancet (London), 2, 1265-1267.

1936. WALTMAN, R., INIQUEZ, F., and INIQUEZ, E.S. (1972) 'Placental transfer of ethanol and its elimination at term.' American Journal of Obstetrics and Gynecology, 40, 180-185.

1937. WARBURTON, D., SUSYER, M., STEIN, Z., and KLINE, J. (1978) 'Genetic and epidemiologic investigations of spontaneous abortion: Relevance to clinical practice.' American Journal of Epidemiology, 108, page ? (abstract).

1938. WARNER, R.H., and ROSETT, H.L. (1975) 'The effects of drinking on offspring: An historical survey of the American and British literature.' Journal of Studies on Alcohol, 36, 1395-1420.

1939. WARREN, K.R. (1977) 'Critical review of the fetal alcohol syndrome.' Presented at the NIAAA Press Conference, Washington, D.C.

1940. WEATHERSBEE, P.S., and LODGE, J.R. (1978) 'A review of ethanol's effects on the reproductive process.' Journal of Reproductive Medicine, 21, 63-78.

1941. WEATHERSBEE, P.S., and LODGE, J.R. (1979) 'Alcohol, caffeine, and nicotine as factors in pregnancy.' Postgraduate Medicine, 66, 165-167, 170-171.

1942. WEBSTER, W.S., LIPSON, A.H., and WALSH, D.A. (1980) 'Teratogenesis of acute alcohol exposure in mice.' Australian Paediatric Journal, 16, 214 (abstract).

1943. WEBSTER, W.S., WALSH, D.A., and LIPSON, A.H. (1980) 'Teratogenesis of acute alcohol exposure in mice.' Teratology, 21, 73A-74A (abstract).

1944. WEBSTER, W.S., WALSH, D.A., LIPSON, A.H., and MC EWEN, S.E. (1980) 'Teratogenesis after acute alcohol exposure in inbred and outbred mice.' Neurobehavioral Toxicology, 2, 227-234.

1945. WEICHSELBAUM, A., and KYRLE, J. (1911) 'Über die Veranderungen der Hoden bei chronischem Alkoholismus.' ['On the changes in the testicles in chronic alcoholism.'] Sitzungsberichte der Akademie der Wissenschaften in Wien (Mathematisch-naturwissenschaftliche Klasse), 120, 56-66.

1946. WEINBERG, J., and GALLO, P.V. (1980) 'Pituitary-adrenal activity in rats prenatally exposed to ethanol.' Paper presented at the International Society for Developmental Psychobiology, Cincinnati, Ohio (November 8).

1947. WEINBERG, J., and GALLO, P.V. (1981) 'Pituitary-adrenal activity following prenatal ethanol exposure: Effects in pregnant females and their offspring.' Teratology, 24, 58A (abstract).

1948. WEINER, L., ROSETT, H.L., and EDELEN, K.C. (1979) 'A brief history of alcohol consumption as part of the prenatal clinic evaluation.' Alcoholism: Clinical and Experimental Research, 3, 200 (abstract).

1949. WEINER, S.G., SHOEMAKER, W., and BLOOM, F.E. (1979) 'Inter-
       action of alcohol and nutrition during gestation: Influence
       on maternal and offspring development in the rat.' Paper
       presented at the International Society for Developmental
       Psychobiology, Atlanta, Georgia (November).

1950. WELLER, C.V. (1916) 'Histological studies of the testes of
       guinea pigs showing lead blastophthoria.' Proceedings
       of the Society for Experimental Biology and Medicine,
       14, 14.

1951. WELLER, C.V. (1921) 'Testicular changes in acute alcoholism in
       man and their relationship to blastophthoria.' Proceedings
       of the Society for Experimental Biology, 19, 131-132.

1952. WELLER, C.V. (1930) 'Degenerative changes in the male germinal
       epithelium in acute alcoholism and their possible relation-
       ship to blastophthoria.' American Journal of Pathology,
       6, 1-18.

1953. WEST, J.R., BLACK, A.C., JR., ALKANA, R.L., and REIMANN, P.C.
       (1979) 'Polydactyly induced by prenatal exposure to eth-
       anol.' Anatomical Record, 193, 718 (abstract).

1954. WEST, J.R., BLACK, A.C., JR., REIMANN, P.C., and ALKANA, R.L.
       (1981) 'Polydactyly and polysyndactyly induced by prenatal
       exposure to ethanol.' Teratology, 24, 13-18.

1955. WEST, J.R., HODGES, C.A., and BLACK, A.C., JR. (1981) 'Abnormal
       neuronal connections in the rat brain following prenatal ex-
       posure to ethanol.' Alcoholism: Clinical and Experimental
       Research, 5, 171 (abstract).

1956. WEST, J.R., HODGES, C.A., and BLACK, A.C., JR. (1981) 'Prenatal
       exposure to ethanol alters the organization of hippocampal
       mossy fibers in rats.' Science, 211, 957-959.

1957. WEST, J.R., SANDQUIST, D., BRUNKO, A.M., COHEN, G.A., HODGES, C.A.,
       and BLACK, A.C., JR. (1980) 'Effects of prenatal ethanol
       exposure on the development of the cyclic GMP response of rat
       hippocampus to muscarinic cholinergic stimulation.' Alco-
       holism: Clinical and Experimental Research, 4, 232 (ab-
       stract).

1958. WESTFELT, G. (1880) 'Om alkoholmissbrukets inflytande pa af-
       kommen och slägtet.' ['On the effects of alcoholism on the
       offspring and species of man.']. Svensk Lakaresallskapets
       NyaHandl Series II, Del VII 2, 168-207.

1959. WESTLING, A. (1954) 'On the correlation of the consumption of
       alcoholic drinks with some sexual phenomena of Finnish male
       students.' International Journal of Sexology, 7, 109-115.

1960. WEYGANDT, W. (1906) 'Über Idiote.' ['Regarding idiots.'] Samm-
       lung zwangloser Abhandlunger aus dem Gebiete der Nerven- und
       Geisteskrankheiten (Halle-an-der-Salle), 6, 186.

1961. WHALLEY, L.J. (1978) 'Sexual adjustment of male alcoholics.' Acta Psychiatrica Scandinavica (Copenhagen), 58, 281-298.

1962. WHALLEY, L.J., and MC GUIRE, R.J. (1978) 'Measuring sexual attitudes.' Acta Psychiatrica Scandinavica (Copenhagen), 58, 299-314.

1963. WIEDEMANN, H.-R., DIBBERN, H., and GROSSE, F.R. (1977) 'Embryofetales Alkoholsyndrom.' ['Fetal alcohol syndrome.'] Medizinische Welt (Stuttgart), 28, 874-875.

1964. WIENER, S.G. (1980) 'Considerations in the design of animal models of FAS.' Paper presented at the International Society for Developmental Psychobiology, Cincinnati, Ohio (November 8).

1965. WIENER, S.G. (1980) 'Nutritional considerations in the design of animal models of the fetal alcohol syndrome.' Neurobehavioral Toxicology, 2, 175-179.

1966. WIENER, S.G. (1980) 'Nutritional and environmental considerations in the design of drug studies during pregnancy.' Teratology, 21, 75A (abstract).

1967. WIENER, S.G., SHOEMAKER, W.J., KODA, L.Y., and BLOOM, F.E. (1981) 'Interaction of ethanol and nutrition during gestation: Influence on maternal and offspring development in the rat.' Journal of Pharmacology and Experimental Therapeutics, 216, 572-579.

1968. WILLIAMS, B. (1979) 'The effect of maternal alcohol consumption during pregnancy.' Journal of the Medical Association of Georgia, 68, 805-809.

1969. WILLIAMS, K.H. (1976) 'An overview of sexual problems in alcoholism.' In: Sexual Counseling for Persons with Alcohol Problems: Proceedings of a Workshop. Ed. J. Newman. Western Pennsylvania Institute of Alcohol Studies, University of Pittsburgh, p. 1.

1970. WILMOT, R. (1981) 'Sexual drinking and drift.' Journal of Drug Issues (Winter), 1-16.

1971. WILSNACK, S.C. (1973) 'Sex role identity in female alcoholism.' Journal of Abnormal Psychology, 82, 253-261.

1972. WILSNACK, S.C. (1974) 'The effects of social drinking on women's fantasy.' Journal of Personality, 42, 43-61.

1973. WILSNACK, S.C. (1976) 'The impact of sex roles on women's alcohol use and abuse.' In: Alcoholism Problems in Women and Children. Ed. M. Greenblatt and M.A. Schuckit. New York: Grune and Stratton, pp. 37-63.

1974. WILSNACK, S.C. (1981) 'Alcohol, sexuality, and reproductive
          dysfunction in women.' In: Fetal Alcohol Syndrome. Vol-
          ume 2: Human Studies. Ed. E.L. Abel. Boca Raton, Florida:
          CRC Press (in press).

1975. WILSNACK, S.C., and WILSNACK, R.W. (1979) 'Sex roles and adoles-
          cent drinking.' In: Youth, Alcohol, and Social Policy.
          Ed. H.T. Blane and M.E. Chafetz. New York: Plenum Press,
          pp. 183-227.

1976. WILSON, A.L., KING, G.J., and FRIAS, J.L. (1980) 'A cephalo-
          metric study of children with the fetal alcohol syndrome.'
          American Journal of Human Genetics, 32, 137A (abstract).

1977. WILSON, G.S. (1980) 'Alcohol and pregnancy don't mix!' [Let-
          ter.] Texas Medicine, 76, 7.

1978. WILSON, G.T. (1977) 'Alcohol and human sexual behavior.' Be-
          havior Research and Therapy (Oxford), 15, 239-252.

1979. WILSON, G.T., and LAWSON, D.M. (1976) 'Effects of alcohol on
          sexual arousal in women.' Journal of Abnormal Psychology,
          85, 489-497.

1980. WILSON, G.T., and LAWSON, D.M. (1976) 'Expectancies, alcohol,
          and sexual arousal in male social drinkers.' Journal of
          Abnormal Psychology, 85, 587-594.

1981. WILSON, G.T., and LAWSON, D.M. (1978) 'Expectancies, alcohol,
          and sexual arousal in women.' Journal of Abnormal Psychol-
          ogy, 87, 358-367.

1982. WILSON, G.T., LAWSON, D.M., and ABRAMS, D.B. (1978) 'Effects
          of alcohol on sexual arousal in male alcoholics.' Journal of
          Abnormal Psychology, 87, 609-616.

1983. WILSON, J. (1978) 'Foetal alcohol syndrome: Considerations for
          action in the U.K.' All Faith's World Alcohol Project Jour-
          nal, 1, 5-7.

1984. WILSON, J. (1980) 'The foetal alcohol syndrome.' Paper pre-
          sented to Short Committee, English House of Commons.

1985. WILSON, J.G. '(1977) 'Embryotoxicity of drugs in man.' In:
          Handbook of Teratology. Volume 1. Ed. J.G. Wilson.
          New York: Plenum Publishing Corporation, pp. 309-355.

1986. WILSON, K.H., LANDESMAN, R., FUCHS, A.-R., and FUCHS, F. (1969)
          'The effect of ethyl alcohol on isolated human myometrium.'
          American Journal of Obstetrics and Gynecology, 104, 436-439.

1987. WISCONSIN JOINT PANEL ON PREVENTION OF FETAL ALCOHOL SYNDROME.
          (1977) 'Prevention, intervention and treatment implications
          for women and children.' Wisconsin Council on Alcohol and
          Other Drug Abuse.

1988. WISNIEWSKI, K., and LUPIN, R.   (1979)   'Fetal alcohol syndrome
            and related CNS problems.' .[Letter.]   Neurology, 29, 1429-
            1430.

1989. WITTI, F.   (1978)   'Alcohol and birth defects.'   FDA Consumer
            Publication, 12, 20-23.   U.S. Department of Health, Ed-
            ucation, and Welfare, No. 78-1047.

1990. WOOD, H.P., and DUFFY, E.L.   (1966)   'Psychosocial factors in
            alcoholic women.'   American Journal of Psychiatry, 123, 341.

1991. WOOD, R.E.   (1977)   'Fetal alcohol syndrome: Its implications
            for dentistry.'   Journal of the American Dental Association,
            95, 596-599.

1992. WOODS, M.   (1916)   'Eight cases of epilepsy in children traced
            to a single intoxication on the part of parents otherwise
            abstainers.'   Paper read before the American Society for the
            Study of Alcohol and Other Narcotics, December 15, 1915.
            Scientific Temperance Journal, 25, 120 (abstract).

1993. WOODSON, P.M., and RITCHEY, S.J.   (1979)   'Effect of maternal
            alcohol consumption on fetal brain cell number and cell
            size.'   Nutrition Reports International, 20, 225-228.

1994. WOODY, C.O., GINTHER, O.J., and POPE, A.L.   (1969)   'Unilateral
            effect of intrauterine injection of alcoholic solutions on
            the corpus luteum of the ewe.'   Journal of Animal Science,
            28, 63-65.

1995. WOOLF, P.   (1979)   'Maternal alcohol ingestion and pregnancy.'
            Midwife, Health Visitor, and Community Nurse, 15, 308, 310.

1996. WOOLLAM, D.H.M.   (1978)   'F.A.S. as an example of mammalian
            teratology.'   All Faith's World Alcohol Project Journal,
            1, n. pag.

1997. WRIGHT, J.M.   (1981)   'Fetal alcohol syndrome: The social work
            connection.'   Health and Social Work, 6, 5-10.

1998. WRIGHT, J.W., FRY, D.E., MERRY, J.   (1976)   'Abnormal hypothal-
            amic-pituitary-gonadal function in chronic alcoholics.'
            British Journal of Addiction (Edinburgh), 71, 211-215.

1999. WUNDERLICH, S.M., BALIGA, B.S., and MUNRO, H.N.   (1979)   'Rat
            placental protein synthesis and peptide hormone secretion in
            relation to malnutrition from protein deficiency or alcohol
            administration.'   Journal of Nutrition, 109, 1534-1541.

Y

2000. YAFFE, S.J. (1978) 'Drugs and pregnancy.' [Editorial.] Clinical Toxicology, 13: 523-533.

2001. YAKUNIN, Y.A., KIPNIS, S.L., BURKOVA, A.S., ERMAKOVA, I.A., ZEMLYANSKAYA, Z.K., KAPE, N.S., RYKINA, I.A., and ANDREEVA, T.M. (1978) 'Role of prenatal pathology in the etiology of lesions of the central nervous system in newborn infants and young children.' [In Russian.] Pediatriia (Moscow), 5, 11-15.

2002. YANAI, J. (1981) 'Comparison of early barbiturate and ethanol effects on the CNS.' Substance and Alcohol Actions/Misuse, 2, 79-91.

2003. YANAI, J., and GINSBURG, B.E. (1973) 'The effect of alcohol consumed by parent mice on the susceptibility to audiogenic seizure and the open-field behavior of their offspring.' Behavior Genetics, 3, 418.

2004. YANAI, J., and GINSBURG, B.E. (1973) 'The effect of early input of ethanol on mice on their susceptibility to audiogenic seizures.' Paper presented at the Third Annual Meeting of the Society for Neuroscience, San Diego, California.

2005. YANAI, J., and GINSBURG, B.E. (1976) 'Audiogenic seizures in mice whose parents drank alcohol.' Journal of Studies on Alcohol, 37, 1564-1571.

2006. YANAI, J., and GINSBURG, B.E. (1976) 'Long-term effects of early ethanol on predatory behavior in inbred mice.' Physiological Psychology, 4, 409-411.

2007. YANAI, J., and GINSBURG, B.E. (1977) 'A developmental study of ethanol effect on behavior and physical development in mice.' Alcoholism: Clinical and Experimental Research, 1, 325-333.

2008. YANAI, J., and GINSBURG, B.E. (1977) 'Long term reduction of male agonistic behavior in mice following early exposure to ethanol.' Psychopharmacology (Berlin), 52, 31-34.

2009. YANAI, J., and GINSBURG, B.E. (1979) 'The relative contribution of pre- and neonatal ethanol administration to changes in mice behavior.' Archives Internationales de Pharmacodynamie et de Thérapie, 241, 235-244.

2010. YANAI, J., GINSBURG, B.E., and VINOPAL, B. (1976) 'Comparison of early effects of ethanol on agonistic behavior in inbred strains of mice.' Behavior Genetics, 6, 122-123.

2011. YANAI, J., SZE, P.Y., and GINSBURG, B.E. (1975) 'Differential induction of behavioral and metabolic changes by ethanol during early development.' Behavior Genetics, 5, 111-112.

2012. YANAI, J., SZE, P.Y., and GINSBURG, B.E. (1975) 'Effects of aminergic drugs and glutamic acid on audiogenic seizures induced by early exposure to ethanol.' Epilepsia, 16, 67-71.

2013. YANAI, J., and TABAKOFF, B. (1980) 'Altered sensitivity to ethanol following prenatal exposure to barbiturate.' Psychopharmacology (Berlin), 68, 301-303.

2014. YAVKIN, V.M. (1978) 'Effects of parental alcoholism on the clinical manifestations of mental retardation in children.' Alcoholism, 14, 97-106.

2015. YESSIAN, N., and NOBLE, E.P. (1981) 'In vitro testosterone synthesis by rat testes following chronic alcohol administration.' Federation Proceedings, 40, 825 (abstract).

2016. YLIKAHRI, R.H. (1978) 'Acute effects of alcohol on anterior pituitary secretion of tropic hormones.' Journal of Clinical Endocrinology and Metabolism, 46, 715-721.

2017. YLIKAHRI, R.H., HUTTUNEN, M.O., and HÄRKÖNEN, M. (1980) 'Hormonal changes during alcohol intoxication and withdrawal.' Pharmacology, Biochemistry, and Behavior, 13, 131-137.

2018. YLIKAHRI, R.H., HUTTUNEN, M.O., HÄRKÖNEN, M., SEUDERLING, U., ONIKKI, S., KARONEN, S.-L., and ADLERCREUTZ, H. (1974) 'Low plasma testosterone values in men during hangover.' Journal of Steroid Biochemistry (Oxford), 5, 655-658.

2019. YOUCHA, G. (1978) A Dangerous Pleasure. New York: Hawthorne Books.

Z

2020. ZASSHI, J. (1980 'Pregnancy and alcohol drinking.' Japanese Journal for Midwives, 34, 47-52.

2021. ZEINER, A.R., and KEGG, P.S. (1979) 'Women and alcohol: Varying effects during the menstrual cycle.' Alcohol Technical Reports, 8, 18-20.

2022. ZEINER, A.R., and KEGG, P.S. (1980) 'Menstrual cycle and oral contraceptive effects on alcohol pharmacokinetics in Caucasian females.' Alcoholism: Clinical and Experimental Research, 4, 233 (abstract).

2023. ZERVOUDAKIS, I.A., KRAUSS, A., and FUCHS, F. (1980) 'Infants of mothers treated with ethanol for premature labor.' American Journal of Obstetrics and Gynecology, 137, 713-718.

2024. ZIPPER, J., MEDEL, M., and PRAGER, R. (1968) 'Alterations in fertility induced by unilateral intrauterine instillation of cytotoxic compounds in rats.' American Journal of Obstetrics and Gynecology, 101, 971-978.

2025. ŽIŽKA, J., BALÍČEK, P., POLÁK, J., HAK, J., and LICHÝ, J. (1978) 'Alkoholová embryopatie: Syndrom poškozeni plodu při nadměrném požívání alkoholu v průběhu těhotenství.' ['Alcohol embryopathy: Syndrome of embryonic damage due to heavy alcohol consumption during pregnancy.'] Československa Pediatrie (Prague), 33: 540-542.

2026. ZLATNICK, F.J., and FUCHS, F. (1972) 'A controlled study of ethanol in threatened premature labor.' American Journal of Obstetrics and Gynecology, 112, 610-612.

Addendum

A

2027. Anonymous. (1981) 'That matcho image.' The Bottom Line 3,
       17-18.

2028. Anonymous. (1981) 'Label campaign in high gear in United States.'
       The Globe, 4, 10-11.

2029. Anonymous. (1981) 'Survey shows high awareness on risks during
       pregnancy.' Discus News Letter, December, 3.

2030. Anonymous (1981) 'Alcohol and your unborn baby.' AARN Newsletter,
       36, 1-2.

2031. Arsenault, R. and Kirouac, G. (1981) 'Effect of ethanol ad-
       ministration during pregnancy on the learning of the
       Hebb Williams maze in the rat.' Canadian Journal of
       Psychology, 35, 356-360.

B

2032.   Barnes, D. E. 'The effects of prenatal ethanol consumption.
        In Goldberg, L. (ed.). Reviews of Toxicology, CRC Press,
        Boca Raton, Florida, in press.

2033.   Barnes, D. E. and Walker, D. W. (1980) 'Neuronal loss in hippo-
        campus induced by prolonged ethanol ingestion in rats.
        Neuroscience Society Abstracts 6, 47.

2034.   Barrison, I. G., Wright, J. T. and Murray-Lyon, I. M. (1981)
        'The hazards of moderate drinking during pregnancy.'
        British Journal on Alcohol and Alcoholism 16, 188-199.

2035.   Bartolome, J. V., Schanberg, S. M. and Slotkin, T. A. (1981)
        'Premature development of cardiac sympathetic neurotrans-
        mission in the fetal alcohol syndrome.' Life Sciences
        28, 571-576.

2036.   Beagle, W. S. (1981) 'Fetal alcohol syndrome: A review.'
        Journal of the American Dietary Association, 79, 274-276.

2037.   Bonds, D., Anderson, S. and Meschia, G. (1980) 'Transplacental
        diffusion of ethanol under steady state conditions.'
        Journal of Developmental Physiology, 2, 409-416.

2037a. Bujdos, O. G., Bergou, J. and Somogyi, E. (1980) 'Health
        defects in children of chronic alcoholics revealed
        by anthropological studies.' Morphologie, Igazsagugyi
        Orvosi Sz 20, 30-35.

2037b. Bush, P. J. (1980) 'Drugs Alcohol and Sex.' Richard Marek
        Publishers, New York.

C

2038.   Castro-Magana, M., Collipp, P. J., Chen, S. Y., Amin, C. S. and Maddaiah, V. T. (1978) 'Zinc levels in one case of fetal alcohol syndrome.' Pediatric Research 12, 515.

2039.   Chasnoff, I. J., Diggs, G. and Schnoll, S. H. (1981) 'Fetal alcohol effects and maternal cough syrup abuse.' American Journal of Diseases of Children 135, 968-971.

2040.   Cobb, C. F., Van Thiel, D. H., and Ennis, M. F. (1978) 'Acetaldehyde and ethanol are testicular toxins.' Gastroenterology, 75, 958.

2041.   Crothers, T. D. (1911) 'Inebriety.' Harvey Publishing Company: Cincinnatti, Ohio.

D

2042. Dalterio, S., Bartke, A., Blum, K. and Sweeney, C. (1981)
       'Marihuana and alcohol: Perinatal effects on development
       of male reproductive functions in mice.' Progress in
       Biochemical Pharmacology, 18, 143-154.

2043. Dening, F. C. (1981) 'Alcohol and the unborn child.'
      Midwives Chronicle and Nursing Notes, 94, 196.

2046. Dubin, N. H., Blake, D. A., Parmley, T. H., Conner, E. A., Cox,
       R. T. and King, T. M. (1978) 'Intrauterine ethanol-induced
       termination of pregnancy in cynomolgus monkeys (Macaca
       fascicularis).' American Journal of Obstetrics and
       Gynecology 132, 783-789.

2047. Dumas, R. M. and Haddad, R. (1981) 'Teratology of ethanol in
       the ferret.' Paper presented at Stanford University
       June 25-26.

2048. Dumas, R. M. and Haddad, R. 'Teratology of ethanol in the
       ferret.' Fundamental and Applied Toxicology, in press.

2049. Dumas, R. M., Haddad, R., Rabe, A. and Lee, M. H. (1981)
       'Use of the ferret for ethanol studies. American
       Association for Laboratory Animal Science, 80-4, 7.

E

2050.   Eckardt, M., Harford, T., Kaelber, C., Parker, E., Rosenthal, L.
        Ryback, R., Salmoiraghi, G., Vanderveen, E., and Warren, K.
        (1981) 'Health hazards associated with alcohol consumption.'
        Journal of the American Medical Association 246, 648-666.

2051.   Eisenberg, J. (1977). 'Zur Biochemie und Klinik der alckoholischen
        Leberschadigung. Zitiert nach.' Gynakologische Praxis
        1, 599-610.

2052.   Erb, L. and Andresen, B. D. (1980) 'Hyperactivity: A possible
        consequence of maternal alcohol consumption.' Pediatric
        Nursing, 7, 30-33, 51.

F

2053. Feifer, M. (1981) 'Don't start your baby on the drink.' Forum, 12, 1-6.

2054. Ficher, M. and Levitt, D. R. (1980) 'Testicular dysfunction and sexual impotence in the alcoholic rat.' Journal of Steroid Biochemistry, 13, 1089-1095.

2055. Finnegan, L. P. (1981) 'The effects of narcotics and alcohol on pregnancy and the newborn.' Annals of the New York Academy of Sciences 362, 136-157.

2056. Finucane, B. T. (1980) 'Difficult intubation associated with the foetal alcohol syndrome.' Canadian Anesthesiology Society Journal 27, 574-575.

2057. Fisher, S. E., Atkinson, M., Holzman, I., David, R. and Van Thiel, D. H. (1981) 'Effect of ethanol upon placental uptake of amino acids.' Progress in Biochemical Pharmacology, 18, 216-223.

2058. Fitzsimons, R. B. (1981) 'Drunk infant.' Pediatrics, 68, 751-753.

2059. Flynn, A., Miller, S. I., Martier, S. S., Golden, N. L., Sokol, R. J. and Villano, B. C. (1981) 'Zinc status of pregnant alcoholic women: A determinant of fetal outcome.' Lancet, 1, 572-573.

2059. Fuchs, A. R. and Fuchs, F. (1974) 'Possible mechanisms of the inhibition of labor by ethanol.' In Josimovich, J. B. (ed.) Uterine Contraction--Side Effects of Steroidal Contraceptives. J. Wiley and Sons: New York, 287-300.

G

2060. Godlewski, J. (1980) 'Problematyka alkoholowa w seksuologii.'
       ('Alcohol problems in sexology.') <u>Problemy</u> <u>Alkoholizmu</u>,
       <u>27</u>, 7-8.

H

2061.   Handicapped Children Fund. (1981) 'Should I Drink?'
        ALFAWAP Trust Fund: London, England.

2062.   Harris, J. M., Tewari, S., and Noble, E. P. (1980) 'The effects of
        chronic ethanol ingestion on rat testicular protein
        synthesis.' Federation Proceedings, 39, 745.

2063.   Heine, M. W. (1981) 'Alcoholism and reproduction.' Progress
        in Biochemical Pharmacology, 18, 75-82.

I

2064. Iosub, S., Fuchs, M., Bingol, N. and Gromisch, D. S. (1981)
      'Fetal alcohol syndrome revisited.' *Pediatrics*, 68,
      475-479.

K

2065.   Kamath, S. H. and Waziri, R. (1978) 'The progeny of alcoholic
        rats.' Alcoholism: Clinical and Experimental Research,
        2, 216.

2066.   Karim, S. M. M. and Sharma, S. D. (1971) 'The effect of ethyl
        alcohol on prostaglandins E_2 and F_2 induced uterine
        activity in pregnant women.' Journal of Obstetrics
        and Gynecology of the British Commonwealth, 78, 251-254.

2067.   Karlsson, G. B. and Sundstrom-Feigenberg, K. (1981) 'Klartext
        fran socialstyrel sen om alkohol och graviditet?'
        ('Plain talk from the National social welfare board on
        alcohol and pregnancy?') Lakartindningen, 78, 929.

2068.   Kaufman, M. H. and Woollam, D. H. M. (1981) 'The passage to
        the fetus and liquor amnii of ethanol administered
        orally to the pregnant mouse.' British Journal of
        Experimental Pathology, 62, 357-361.

2068à. Kennedy, L. A. and Persaud, T. V. N. (1981) 'Teratological
        evaluation of ethanol, pentobarbital and combination
        of these, in the rat.' Teratology, 17, 40A.

L

2069.   Lauersen, N. H., Merkatz, I. R., Tejani, N., Wilson, K. H.,
        Roberson, A., Mann, L. I. and Fuchs, F. (1977)
        'Inhibition of premature labor: A multicenter comparison
        of ritodrine and ethanol.' American Journal of Obstetrics
        and Gynecology 127, 837-845.

2070.   Lin, G. W. J. (1981) 'Fetal malnutrition: A possible cause
        of the fetal alcohol syndrome.' Progress in Biochemical
        Pharmacology 18, 115-121.

2071.   Lochry, E. A., Randall, C. L., Goldsmith, A. A. and Sutker, P. B.
        'The effects of acute alcohol exposure during selected
        days of gestation in C3H mice.' Neurobehavioral
        Toxicology and Teratology, in press.

2072.   Loser, H. (1981) 'Human alcohol embryopathy and changes at the
        cardiovascular system.' Teratology, 24, 29A-29B.

2073.   Lyons, J. P., Russell, M. and Brown, J. (1980) 'Computer-aided
        alcoholism diagnosis in obstetric and gynecologic settings.'
        Paper presented at 11th Annual Medical-Scientific Conference
        of the National Alcoholism Forum, Seattle, Washington,
        May 2-4.

M

2074.   Majewski, F. (1981)'Teratogenic risk due to alcohol consumption,
         experimental and clinical experiences.' Teratology, 24,
         30A-31A.

2074a.   Messiha, F. S. (1981) 'Subcellular fractionation of alcohol
         and aldehyde dehydrogenase in the rat testicles.'
         Progress in Biochemical Pharmacology, 18, 155-166.

2074b.   Miller, M., Israel, J. and Cuttone, J. (1981) 'Fetal alcohol
         syndrome.' Journal of Pediatric Ophthalmology and
         Strabismus, 18, 6-15.

N

2075.   Nestler, V., Spohr, H. I. and Steinhausen, H. C. (1981)
         'Studies on alcohol embryopathy.' Monatsschrift fur
         Kinderheilkunde, 129, 404-409.

2075a.   Neugut, R. H. (1981) 'Epidemiological appraisal of the
         literature on the fetal alcohol syndrome in humans.'
         Early Human Development, 5, 411-429.

O

2076. Obe, G. (1980) 'Mutagenic activity of ethanol.' In
       Ericksson, K., Sinclair, J. D. and Kiianmaa, K. (eds.).
       Animal Models in Alcohol Research. Academic Press:
       New York, 377-391.

2077. Obe, G., Gobel, D., Engelan, H., Herha, J. and Natarajan, A. T.
       'Chromosomal aberrations in peripheral lymphocytes of
       alcoholics.' Mutation Research 73, 377-386.

2078. Osztovics, M., Igali, S., Antal, A. and Veghelyi, P. (1980)
       'Alcohol is not mutagenic.' Mutation Research, 74, 247.

P

2079. Patwardhan, R., Schenker, S., Henderson, G., Abou-mourad, N. and Hoyumpa, A. (1981) 'Short-term and long-term ethanol administration inhibits the placental uptake and transport of valine in rats.' Journal of Laboratory Clinical Medicine, 98, 251-262.

2080. Persaud, T. V. N. and Anders, K. 'Compensatory embryonic development in the rat following maternal treatment with ethanol. Anat. Anz. 148, 375-383.

2081. Persaud, T. V. N. and Anders, K. 'Effects of alcohol on the early rat embryo.' Anatomical Record, 196, 8A.

2082. Persaud, T. V. N. and Kennedy, L. A. 'Prenatal toxicity of alcohol in the rat.' Proceedings of the Canadian Federation for Biology Society, 20, 18.

2083. Pikkarainen, P. H. (1971) 'Metabolism of ethanol and acetaldehyde in perfused human fetal liver.' Life Sciences 10, 1359-1364.

2084. Pikkarainen, P. H. and Raiha, N. C. R. (1967) 'Development of alcohol dehydrogenase activity in the human liver.' Pediatric Research, 1, 165-168.

2085. Pratt, O. (1981) 'Alcohol and the woman of childbearing age-- A public health problem.' British Journal of Addiction, 76, 383-390.

2086. Puig, M., Arce, A., Juana, R., Leandro, S. V. and Villa-Elizaga, I. (1980) "Sindrome de alcohol fetal.' Revista De Medicina De La Universidad De Navarra, 23, 34-44.

R

2087.   Randall, C. L. (1980) 'Fetal alcohol syndrome: Overview for
        medical professionals.' Alcohol and Drug Abuse Newsletter,
        University of Illinois, 1, 2-10.

2088.   Randall, C. 'Alcohol as a teratogen in animals.' In
        National Institute on Alcohool Abuse and Alcoholism.
        Biomedical Processes and Consequences of Alcohol Use.
        National Institute on Alcohol Abuse and Alcoholism:
        Rockville, Maryland, in press.

2089.   Randall, C. L., Burling, T. A., Lochry, E. A. and Sutker, P. B.
        'The effect of paternal alcohol consumption on fetal
        development in mice.' Drug and Alcohol Dependence, in press.

2090.   Ristow, H. and Obe, G. 'Acetaldehyde induces cross-links in
        DNA and causes sister chromatid exchanges in human cells.'
        Mutation Research, 58, 115-119.

2091.   Rose, J. C., Strandhoy, J. W. and Meis, P. J. (1981) 'Acute
        and chronic effects of maternal ethanol administration
        on the ovine maternal-fetal unit.' Progress in Biochemical
        Pharmacology, 18, 1-14.

2091a. Royce, J. E. (1981) 'Alcohol Problems and Alcoholism
        A Comprehensive Survey.' New York: The Free Press.

S

2092.   Salaspuro, M. P. and Lieber, C. S. (1981) "Comparison of the
        detrimental effects of chronic alcohol intake in humans
        and animals.' In Eriksson, Sinclair, J. D. and Kiianmaa, K.
        (eds.). Animal Models in Alcohol Research. Academic Press:
        New York, 359-376.

2093.   Samson, H. H., Grant, K. A., Coggan, S. and Sachs, V. M.
        'Ethanol induced microcephaly in the neonatal rat: Occurrence
        without withdrawal.' Neurobehavioral Toxicology and
        Teratology, in press.

2094.   Sandor, S. (1981) 'The effect of ethanol upon early development
        in mice and rats. III. In vivo effects of acute ethanol
        intoxication upon implantation and early postimplantation
        stages in mice.' Revue Roumaine de Morphologie, D'embryologie
        et de Physiologie, 27, 117-122.

2095.   Sandor, S., Checiu, M., Fazakas-Todea, I. and Garban, Z. (1980)
        'The effect of ethanol upon early development in mice and
        rats. I. In vivo effects upon preimplantation and early
        postimplantation stages.' Revue Roumaine de Morphologie
        D'embryologie et de Physiologie, 26, 265-274.

2096.   Sasaki, S. (1981) 'Fetal alcohol syndrome.' Josanpu Zasshi,
        35, 315-318.   (In Japanese).

2097.   Schmatolla, E. (1975) 'Retino-tectal course of optic nerves in
        cyclopic and synophthalmic Zebrafish embryos.'
        Anatomical Record, 180, 377-384.

2098.   Shanske, A. L. and Kazi, R. (1980) 'Prevelance of the fetal
        alcohol syndrome in a developmental clinic population.'
        American Journal of Human Genetics, 32, 128A.

2099.   Shaywitz, S. E., Caparulo, B. K. and Hodgson, E. S. (1981)
'Developmental language disability as a consequence
of prenatal exposure to ethanol.' Pediatrics, 68, 850-
855.

2100.   Shuman, R. M., Adickes, E. D., Jacobsen, J and Kader, F. J.
(1981) 'Fetal alcohol myopathy.' Laboratory Investigation,
44, 7P.

2101.   Sitzmann, F. C. (1980) 'Die Alkohol-embryofetopathie.'
('Alcohol embryofetopathy.')   Zeitschrift fuer Allege-
meinmedizin, 56, 985-989.

2102.   Stromland, K. (1981) 'Eyeground malformations in the fetal
alcohol syndrome.' Neuropediatrics, 12, 97-98.

2103.   Stromland, K. (1981) 'Malformations of the eyes in fetal
alcohol syndrome.' Acta Ophthalmology, 59, 445-446.

2104.   Sundstrom-Feigenberg, K., Sjogren, I., Edvardsson, N. and
Olsson, S. B. (1981) 'Missbruk under graviditet och i
barnfamiljen.' ('Abuse during pregnancy and in the
child's family.') Lakartidningen, 78, 105-107.

2105.   Takashima, H., Bab, K., Kunugida, F. (1978) 'One family of the
        fetal alcohol syndrome in Japan.' (in Japanese).
        Alcohol Research, 13, 102-103.

2106.   Takashima, H. (1979) 'The fetal alcohol syndrome in Japan.'
        (In Japanese). Japanese Medical Journal, 2897, 27-30.

2107.   Tanaka, H., Arima, M. and Suzuki, N. (1981) 'The fetal alcohol
        syndrome in Japan.' Brain and Development, 3, 305-311.

2108.   Taylor, A. N., Branch, B. J., and Kokka, N. (1981) 'Neuro-
        endocrine effects of fetal alcohol exposure.'
        Progress in Biochemical Pharmacology, 18, 99-110.

2109.   Thadani, P. V. (1981) 'Fetal alcohol syndrome: Neurochemical
        and endocrinological abnormalities.' Progress in
        Biochemical Pharmacology, 18, 83-98.

2110.   Trotter, T. (1813) 'An Essay, Medical, Philosophical, and
        Chemical on Drunkenness, and Its Effects on the Human
        Body.' Anthony Finley: Philadelphia.

2111.   Tumbleson, M. E., Dexter, J. D. and Middleton, C. C. (1981)
        'Voluntary ethanol consumption by female offspring from
        alcoholic and control Sinclair (S-1) miniature dams.'
        Progress in Biochemical Pharmacology, 18, 179-189.

V

2112.   Van Thiel, D. H., Gavalair, J. S., Herman, G. B., Lester, R.,
        Smith, W. I. and Gay, V. L. (1980) 'An evaluation of the
        respective roles of liver disease and malnutrition
        in the pathogenesis of the hypogonadism seen in alcoholic
        rats.' Gastroenterology, 79, 533-538.

2113.   Varma, S. Sharma, K. and Bharat, B. (1981) 'Fetal alcohol
        syndrome.' Progress in Biochemical Pharmacology, 18,
        122-129.

2114.   Valimaki, M. and Ylikahri, R. (1981) 'Alcohol and sex
        hormones.' Scandinavian Journal of Clinical and
        Laboratory Investigation, 41, 99-105.

2115.   Volk, B., Maletz, J., Tiedemann, M., Mall, G., Klein, C. and
        Berlet, H. H. (1981) 'Impaired maturation of purkinje cells in
        fetal alcohol syndrome of the rat. Light and electron micro-
        scopic investigations.' Acta Neuropathologica, 54, 19-29.

2116.   Volk, B., Maletz, J., Tiedemann, M., Ilzenhofer, H. and Berlet,
        H. H. (1980) 'Impaired development of synaptic junctions of
        rat brain in fetal alcohol syndrome. Morphological and
        biochemical studies. In Brzin, M., Sket, D., and Bachelard,
        H. (eds.). Proceedings of the Third Meeting of the European
        Society of Neurochemistry. Pergamon Press: Oxford, 407.

2117.   Vorhees, C. V. and Butcher, R. E. (1982) 'Behavioural terato-
        genicity.' In Snell, K. (ed.). Developmental Toxicology.
        Croom Helm Press: London, 247-298.

W

2118.   Watring, W. G., Benson, W. L., Wiebe, R. A. and Vaughn, D. L.
        (1976) 'Intravenous alcohol--A single blind study in the
        prevention of premature delivery: A preliminary report.'
        Journal of Reproductive Medicine, 16, 35-38.

2119.   Wilmot, R. 'Sexual drinking and drift.' Journal of Drug
        Issues, 11, 1-16.

2120.   Wilson, J. (1981) 'The fetal alcohol syndrome.' Public Health,
        95, 129-132.

Subject Index

The numbers in this index refer to entry numbers, not page numbers.

Alcohol and Smoking, Effects of combined use on

    Behavior   1147, 1408.

    Growth retardation 1707

    Stillbirth   673

    See also: Interactions

Amino acids   495, 583, 586, 744, 745, 749, 750, 855, 896, 1003, 1004,

    1005, 1006, 1057, 1208, 1438, 1813, 1932, 2070, 2079.

Anencephaly 455, 456, 458, 1783.

Anoxia/Apnea   337, 594, 783, 859, 998, 1309, 1917.

Arterial pressure   390.

Autopsy studies   360, 366, 367, 691, 844, 901, 1116, 1354, 1817, 1886.

Avoidance learning

    Active   6, 10, 151, 248, 249, 251, 253, 315, 723, 724, 1317, 1641,

        2036.

    Passive 422, 476, 625, 1046, 1484.

Beer   See: Beverage alcohol

Behavioral teratology review   17, 18, 19, 21, 22.

    See also: Reviews

Beverage alcohol   14, 15, 29, 30, 33, 34, 141, 145, 146, 872.

Binge drinking   410, 485, 1175, 1427.

Birth during intoxication   208.

Birth Weight

    Animal studies   6, 32, 35, 58, 59, 106, 249, 252, 253, 302, 315,

        416, 434, 451, 456, 458, 527, 546, 709, 723, 769, 771, 975, 978,

        987, 1042, 1046, 1048, 1149, 1303, 1317, 1331, 1368, 1369, 1377,

        1468, 1484, 1507, 1641, 1642, 1651, 1801, 1810, 1848, 1868, 1922.

    Human studies   1020, 1022, 1024, 1026, 1039, 1138, 1140, 1554.

    Reviews   19, 23, 39.

About the Compiler

ERNEST L. ABEL is a Research Scientist at the Research Institute on Alcoholism in Buffalo, a part of the Division of Alcoholism and Acohol Abuse of the State of New York. He has compiled *A Marihuana Dictionary* (Greenwood Press, 1982) and has written many books on a variety of subjects including *Handwriting on the Wall: Towards a Sociology and Psychology of Graffiti* (Greenwood Press, 1977).